THE GIFT
OF DYSLEXIA

Why Some of the Smartest People
Can't Read . . . and How They Can Learn

THIRD EDITION

Ronald D. Davis
with Eldon M. Braun

Souvenir Press

First published in the USA by Perigee,
an imprint of Penguin Group (USA) Inc.

First British edition published 1995 by Souvenir Press

Second British edition, revised and enlarged,
first published 1997 by Souvenir Press
Reprinted seventeen times.

This third revised edition first published in Great Britain in 2010
by Souvenir Press Ltd, 43 Great Russell Street, London WC1B 3PD

Reprinted 2010, 2011

While the author has made every effort to provide
accurate telephone numbers and Internet addresses at the time of publication,
neither the publisher nor author assumes any responsibility for errors, or for
changes that occur after publication. Further, the publisher does not have
any control over and does not assume any responsibility for author
or third-party websites or their content.

The right of Ronald D. Davis to be identified as the author
of this work has been asserted by him in accordance with the
Copyright, Designs and Patents Act, 1988

ISBN   9780285638730

'Funky Winkerbean' cartoon reprinted with special permission of
North America Syndicate, Inc.
'Self-esteem' cartoon by Koren, copyright © 1992 by
The New Yorker Magazine, Inc.
Davis, Davis Dyslexia Correction, Davis Orientation Counseling, and Davis
Symbol Mastery are registered trademarks owned by Ronald D. Davis.

Interior illustrations by Mia Sutter
Interior photographs by P. Courtney Davis
Computer graphic illustrations by Mark Gittus

Printed in the UK by CPI William Clowes Beccles NR34 7TL

In honor and memory of
Harold Joseph Anderson,
one man who cared

Contents

Foreword

Why is this book important? Because the methods described in it work. Because the techniques can be used to ameliorate a wide variety of symptoms besides reading difficulties—from anxiety to writing difficulties to inability to concentrate. Because it recognizes the unusual gifts and the extraordinary potential of dyslexics. Because it turns the mysteries of orientation and disorientation into practical, life-changing techniques. Because the ability to think in pictures is needed for success in the twenty-first century.

I was introduced to Ron Davis's work 25 years ago, by my dear friend and colleague at the Gifted Development Center, Betty Maxwell. One of our clients enrolled in the Davis Dyslexia Correction Program and returned with enthusiastic stories of the unique methods Ron used and the progress her daughter had made in reading. She had also shared with Ron some of our articles on visual-spatial learners and he immediately recognized that we were on the same wavelength. We were both talking about individuals who were picture-thinkers.

Betty and I had been developing the concept of the visual-spatial learner since the early 1980s. These children think in pictures rather than in words, need hands-on experiences to learn, and often reach conclusions without appearing to take the logical steps. So the directive "show your work" mystifies them. "I just saw it in my head!" doesn't gain any credit on standardized achievement tests.

When we first began studying visual-spatial learners, we thought that they represented a small percentage of the student body. We were surprised when field-testing of our Visual-Spatial Identifier revealed that at least one-third of the regular classroom was strongly visual-spatial. Davis Dyslexia Facilitator Crystal Punch writes that there is a "need for educators to truly understand this visual process, or . . . it oftentimes is diagnosed as something else. . . . It truly is a different learning style just requiring a paradigm shift in learning, learning a visual way."

We recognized that Ron's approach was perfect for those visual-spatial children who struggle to master reading. The main difference between his population and ours was that most of our visual-spatial learners were excellent readers. Why? As we delved into the developmental histories of these children, we noted that the vast majority had taught themselves to read before school age. They had absorbed whole words well in advance of sound/symbol awareness. They had started with stop signs, storefronts, and cereal boxes—images they could visualize. They weren't constrained to having to string together phonemes. Had their first encounter with reading been in the classroom, perhaps they would not have excelled.

We have recommended *The Gift of Dyslexia* to our clients who struggled with decoding words, and we have referred many of them to the Davis Dyslexia Correction Center, as well as to the providers Ron has trained all over the world. We do this because Ron's methods achieve results. One exceptionally gifted boy we sent to work with Ron and his associates gained four grade levels in reading in one week, and he retained that growth over time.

One of Ron's more compelling ideas is that genius does not occur *in spite of* learning disabilities, but *because* of them. He is right. I had the good fortune of meeting Patience Thomson, creator of the Barrington Stoke reading series for reluctant readers, when we both spoke at a conference on visual-spatial learners at Green College, Oxford University, sponsored by the Arts Dyslexia Trust. Patience is the daughter and granddaughter of Nobel Prize winners in physics. Her husband is the son and grandson of Nobel Prize winners in Physics. A family tree of both sides of the family was posted during the conference. Artists and dyslexics are prevalent in these family lines. What is the relationship between dyslexics, artists and geniuses in physics? They all see the world in a unique manner, with greater activation of their right hemispheres. The brain organization that creates dyslexia also enables revolutionary breakthroughs in the complex arena of physics.

Ron lists all of the essential gifts of dyslexics, including greater development of intuition, the ability to perceive multi-dimensionally, vivid imagination, greater curiosity, insightful-ness, the ability to experience thought as reality, heightened awareness of the environment, the ability to think in pictures, and, most important, the ability to alter and create perceptions. These are vital gifts, becoming more and more sought after in the work world in the modern era.

While we are still obsessed in education with the importance of literacy, the future of today's students is dependent on their ability to see the big picture, to predict trends, to read customers, to think outside the box, to see patterns, to inspire collaboration among peers, to empathize, to synthesize information from a variety of sources, and to perceive possibilities from different perspectives. These are the natural talents of dyslexics. And Ron has developed a powerful method that allows them to learn to read efficiently without sacrificing any of these important abilities.

I am honored to write the foreword to this new edition of Ron Davis's *Gift of Dyslexia*, and I feel blessed to know this creative thinker, who has revolutionized our understanding of dyslexia and been such a gift to the special individuals he serves.

Dr. Linda Kreger Silverman

Dr. Linda Kreger Silverman is a licensed psychologist and founder of the Institute for the Study of Advanced Development and its subsidiaries, the Gifted Development Center and Visual-Spatial Resource. She has contributed to more than 300 publications and is the author of Upside-Down Brilliance: The Visual-Spatial Learner *and the textbook* Counseling the Gifted and Talented.

Author's Note

The Gift of Dyslexia is intentionally typeset with larger than normal type and the fewest possible number of hyphens to make it dyslexic-friendly.

Preface

A scene from my life in 1949 . . .

The clock on the classroom wall ticks slower and slower. Tick . . . tick . . . tick . . .

"Please hurry! Please hurry! Please—please—please hurry!" The words are whispered barely aloud by the young boy. Every muscle in his body is tense. His fingers twitch and tremble. His knees, pressed tightly together, quiver and touch the walls of the corner. He rocks slowly back and forth, but is careful not to dislodge the folded white handkerchief, his label of unworthiness, draped like a flag across the top of his head.

"Please—please!" he whispers again. Then he sucks in his breath and winces. But it doesn't help; nothing can. Within minutes it starts, a trickle at first, then all of it. He silently hopes there isn't so much that it makes a puddle on the floor.

He hunches over, pressing his face tight into the corner. His wrists cross into an X in his lap, hoping to hide the wet spot. Now he is glad he won't be leaving the school when the other kids do. Maybe they'll all be gone when he leaves and nobody will see; nobody will tease him. He has hoped this hope at least a hundred times before, but maybe this time he won't hear those awful words:

"Retard!"

"Retard!"

"Look at the retard."

"Retard pissed his pants again."

He is startled by the bell that signals school is out for the day. In the corner, amidst the clatter and clamor of the kids leaving, the boy sits motionless, hoping nobody looks in his direction. If he could be invisible he would be. Not until the room is quiet does he dare move, does he dare make a sound.

As the noise fades, the ticking of the clock accelerates. Tick . . . tick, tick!

Barely aloud, the boy whispers something that only he should hear.

"What did you say?" The loud voice booms right behind him.

If he hadn't already done it, he would be wetting his pants now. He presses into the corner as tightly as he can and tries to be as small as he can be.

One of the hands that put him in the corner grabs his shoulder and pulls him around. "What did you say?" the voice demands.

"I asked God not to make me sit in the corner anymore."

That child's prayer is the sole reason for this book.

Acknowledgments

Even though Eldon Braun and I have our names on this book, we are not its only creators. My wife, Alice, has worked just as hard as either of us to put this book in your hands. In addition to being our editor, she has been the mediator of conflicts, the soother of ruffled feathers and the doctor of bruised egos.

Two others deserve special thanks: Dr. Fatima Ali, who has been the CEO of the Reading Research Council and my mentor since 1981, and Larry J. Rochester, without whose help we would have never gotten started.

Others who have given inspiration, commitment and support include:

Rakaia Ansari
Dr. Richard Blasband
Alease Helmick Davis
Philip Courtney Davis
Sarah Derr
Jim Evers
Bill and Charlotte Foster

Dr. Louis Gann
Jeff Gershow
Dr. Albrecht Giese
Rev. Beth Gray
Dr. Brian Halevie-Goldman
Chris Jackson
Betty Ann and Dehlia Judah
Keith and June Monaghan
Vickie Morgan
Jacqueline Pratt
Dana Rahlmann
Marilyn Rosenthal
Dr. Barry Schwartz
Dr. Joan Smith
Jill Stowell
Dorothy Towner

Finally, my thanks to the thousands of dyslexics who have walked through the doors of the Reading Research Council and to those who continue to show up each week. It is they who are answering my prayer and helping me finally get out of my corner.

PART ONE

What Dyslexia Really Is

FUNKY WINKERBEAN

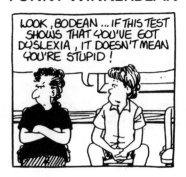

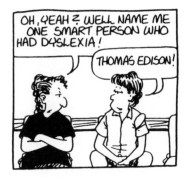

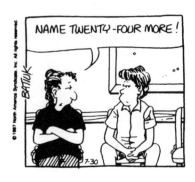

CHAPTER 1

The Underlying Talent

Usually when people hear the word *dyslexia* they think only of reading, writing, spelling and math problems a child is having in school. Some associate it only with word and letter reversals, some only with slow learners. Almost everyone considers it some form of a learning disability, but the learning disability is only one face of dyslexia.

Once, as a guest on a television show, I was asked about the "positive" side of dyslexia. As part of my answer, I listed a dozen or so famous dyslexics. The hostess of the show then commented, "Isn't it amazing that all those people could be geniuses in spite of having dyslexia."

She missed the point. Their genius didn't occur *in spite* of their dyslexia, but *because* of it!

Famous Dyslexics

Hans Christian Andersen	Danny Glover
Harry Belafonte	Whoopi Goldberg
Alexander Graham Bell	Bruce Jenner
John Britten	Jay Leno
George Burns	Greg Louganis
Stephen J. Cannell	General George Patton
Cher	Nelson Rockefeller
Winston Churchill	Charles Schwab
Leonardo da Vinci	Jackie Stewart
Walt Disney	Quentin Tarantino
Albert Einstein	Woodrow Wilson
Henry Ford	W. B. Yeats

Having dyslexia won't make every dyslexic a genius, but it is good for the self-esteem of all dyslexics to know their minds work in exactly the same way as the minds of great geniuses. It is also important for them to know that having a problem with reading, writing, spelling or math doesn't mean they are dumb or stupid. The same mental function that produces a genius can also produce those problems.

The mental function that causes dyslexia is a gift in the truest sense of the word: *a natural ability, a talent.* It is something special that enhances the individual.

Dyslexics don't all develop the same gifts, but they do have certain mental functions in common. Here are the basic abilities all dyslexics share:

1. They can utilize the brain's ability to alter and create perceptions (the primary ability).
2. They are highly aware of the environment.
3. They are more curious than average.
4. They think mainly in pictures instead of words.
5. They are highly intuitive and insightful.
6. They think and perceive multidimensionally (using all the senses).
7. They can experience thought as reality.
8. They have vivid imaginations.

These eight basic abilities, if not suppressed, invalidated or destroyed by parents or the educational process, will result in two characteristics: higher-than-normal intelligence and extraordinary creative abilities. From these the true gift of dyslexia can emerge—the gift of mastery.

The gift of mastery develops in many ways and in many areas. For Albert Einstein, it was physics; for Walt Disney, it was art; for Greg Louganis, it was athletic prowess.

A Paradigm Shift

To change our perspective of dyslexia from disability to gift, we must start with a clear, accurate understanding of what dyslexia really is, and what causes it. Doing this will bring out the positive as well as the negative aspects of the situation and allow us to see how dyslexia develops. Then the idea of correcting it won't seem far-fetched. Going a step beyond correcting the problem, we can also recognize and explore this condition as the gift it truly is.

Before a dyslexic person can fully realize and appreciate the positive side of dyslexia, the negative side should be addressed. That doesn't mean the positive side will not surface until the problems are solved. The gift is always there, even if it isn't recognized for what it is. In fact, many adult dyslexics use the positive side of dyslexia in their life work without realizing it. They just think they have a *knack* for doing something, without realizing their special talent comes from the same mental functions that prevent them from being able to read, write or spell very well.

The most common disabilities of dyslexia occur in reading, writing, spelling or math; but there are many others. Each case of dyslexia is different, because dyslexia is an unintentionally *self-created condition.* No two dyslexics have created it exactly the same.

In order to understand the *gift of dyslexia*, we need to view the learning disability known as dyslexia from a different angle.

Dyslexia is the result of a perceptual talent. In some situations, the talent becomes a liability. The individual doesn't realize this is happening because use of the talent has become integrated into the thought process. It began very early in life and by now seems as natural as breathing.

CHAPTER 2

The Learning Disability

Dyslexia was the first general term used to describe various learning problems. Eventually, these problems were subdivided and categorized to describe different learning disabilities. Because of this, we might call dyslexia the Mother of Learning Disabilities. By now, more than 70 names are used to describe its various aspects.

Originally, researchers thought dyslexic people had some form of brain or nerve damage, or a congenital malfunction that interfered with the mental processes necessary for reading.

Then, in the late 1920s, Dr. Samuel Torrey Orton redefined dyslexia as "cross lateralization of the brain." This meant that the left side of the brain was doing what the right side was normally supposed to do, and the right side was doing the job of the left side. This was only a theory, and before long he decided it was incorrect. Then he introduced a second theory, saying that dyslexia was "mixed hemispheric dominance." This meant that *sometimes* the right side of the brain was doing what the left side was supposed to, and vice versa.

Today there are many different theories of what dyslexia is and what causes it. Most were formulated to explain the symptoms or characteristics of dyslexia—and why the disability occurred.

A New Perspective

The theories and procedures in this book were developed not to explain the nature of the problem, but to explain *why it could be corrected.* The theories were developed during and after the development of the corrective procedures described in the final chapters. Because I used "hindsight," and because I have firsthand experience at being a dyslexic, mine is an entirely different perspective.

This is what I've found out: dyslexia is not the result of brain damage or nerve damage. Nor is it caused by a malformation of the brain, inner ear or eyeballs. Dyslexia is a product of thought and a special way of reacting to the feeling of confusion.

Two Kinds of Thought

It is widely believed that human beings think in two different ways: "verbal conceptualization" and "non-verbal conceptualization."

Verbal conceptualization means thinking with the *sounds* of words. Nonverbal conceptualization means thinking with mental *pictures* of concepts or ideas.

Verbal thought is linear in time. It follows the structure of language. When using it, a person composes mental sentences one word at a time. Verbal thinking occurs at about the same speed as speech. Normal speech has a speed of about 150 words per minute, or 2.5 words per second.

A skilled radio announcer or auctioneer can race along at 200 words per minute. Electronically doctored speech can remain intelligible to an attentive listener at speeds of up to 250 words per minute. This is essentially the maximum limit of verbal conceptualization.

Nonverbal thought is evolutionary. The picture "grows" as the thought process adds more concepts. Nonverbal thought is much faster, possibly thousands of times faster. In fact, it's difficult to understand the nonverbal thinking process because it happens so fast you aren't aware of it when you do it. Usually nonverbal thinking is subliminal, or below conscious awareness.

People think in both verbal and nonverbal modes, but being human, we have a tendency to specialize. Each person will practice one mode as his primary mode of thinking and the other as a secondary mode.

During the period when the learning disability aspect of dyslexia is formed, between the ages of three and thirteen, the potential dyslexic must be primarily a nonverbal thinker—a person who thinks in pictures.

To see how this mode of thinking contributes to the dyslexic's learning disability, we must look at our language. We can consider language a mirror of the thought process. Otherwise language would be far too complicated for anyone to learn.

Language is composed of symbols. Symbols are composed of three parts:

1. What the symbol sounds like
2. What the symbol means
3. What the symbol looks like

When we use verbal conceptualization, we are thinking with the *sounds* of the language. We are actually carrying on an internal monologue of mental statements, questions and answers. Some people verbalize these conceptualizations by talking to themselves out loud. It's a slow process, but one that can make the meaning of a sentence easy to get, even though some of the words may not be fully understood.

Listening to a sentence mentally can aid understanding, because all the symbols (letters and words) don't usually occur in a sequence that makes the meaning of the sentence unfold as it is being read. For instance, you can't tell whether an English sentence is a statement or a question until you get to the end and discover whether it is followed by a period or a question mark—can you?

If we use nonverbal conceptualization, we are thinking

with the meaning of the language by forming mental pictures of its concepts and ideas. The pictures aren't just visual. They are more like three-dimensional, multisensory movies. They change and evolve as a sentence is read. The process is many times faster than verbal conceptualization. But it does present a problem, because some parts of the language are easier to picture as concepts and ideas than others.

Keep in mind that dyslexics have little or no internal monologue, so they do not *hear* what they are reading unless they are reading aloud. Instead, they are composing a mental picture by adding the meaning—or image of the meaning—of each new word as it is encountered.

Two Kinds of Words

Words that describe real things don't cause dyslexics much trouble.

In nonverbal thought, we can think with the word *elephant* easily if we know what an elephant looks like. The animal we call an "elephant" is the literal meaning of the word *elephant.* Seeing its picture is seeing its meaning. We can think with the word *home* if we can picture a place where we once lived. We can think with nouns like *school*, *book*, *paper* and *pencil* as long as we know what they look like. We can think with verbs like *fly*, *sleep*, *view* and the like, because we have seen or experienced the actions the words describe.

11

It is impossible for a nonverbal thinker to think with words whose meanings can't be pictured. Knowing what an *a* looks like doesn't let us think with an *a*. Nor does knowing what an *and* or a *the* looks like allow us to think with those words. Seeing the letters *t-h-e* for the word *the* is not seeing its meaning. The only picture available is the forms of the letters themselves. When we use the picturing process of nonverbal thinking, we are not able to picture the meaning of the word as an object or an action.

If we read a sentence while we are using verbal conceptualization, seeing words like *a*, *and* and *the* won't create a problem, because we know how they sound. We will create a picture of the meaning of a sentence only after we have completed reading the sentence. Even if we don't know the exact meanings of these words, we won't have a problem, because the overall idea of the sentence will be understood after we finish reading it and listen to it mentally.

Reading the same sentence while using nonverbal conceptualization will produce dyslexic symptoms. The picture of the sentence's meaning is evolving as we read. The evolutionary development of the picture being formed by the sentence is stopped each time the meaning of an unknown word cannot be incorporated into the overall picture. The problem will be compounded every time we come across a word whose meaning does not have a corresponding mental picture. We end up with a series of unrelated pictures with blank spots in between.

In nonverbal conceptualization, each time the picture-making process is stopped, the person will experience a feeling of confusion because the picture being composed becomes more incoherent. Using concentration, the reader can push past the blanks and continue, but he will feel more and more confused the further he goes. Eventually he will reach his *threshold of confusion.*

At this point, the person becomes *disoriented.*

Disorientation means that perception of the symbols gets altered and becomes distorted so that reading or writing is difficult or impossible. Ironically, this shifting of perception is the exact mechanism that dyslexics have found useful for recognizing real-life objects and events in their environment before they began learning to read.

CHAPTER 3

Effects of Disorientation

Orientation means knowing where you are in relation to your environment. In terms of perception, it means finding out the facts and conditions of your surroundings and putting yourself in the proper relation to them. When you see, hear and sense the outside world from a particular viewpoint that makes sense to you, you are oriented. An airplane or ship navigator has the job of determining the orientation of a plane or ship to its environment.

Humans orient themselves visually by looking at the world through two eyes. The brain compares the two images the eyes see and uses the difference between them to form a three-dimensional mental image that tells us how far away things are. The ears do the same thing to determine from which direction a sound is coming. This technique is known as triangulation. It works the same way in perception as in navigation.

ceive from visually is not on
cause those are two different
al "screen" in the brain. People
sion that they are looking out
ere behind their eyes.

lind's Eye

erception point from which a
person looks at mental images and thoughts. If you
close your eyes and look at an imaginary mental
picture, this point of perception is where you are
looking from, or what you are using in order to look.
It is not the same as the visual perception point, but
works on the same basic principle as vision: something
is looking at something else. This "epicenter of
perception" is what I call "the mind's eye." When it
shifts, it causes all the physical perceptions to disorient.
This is fully explained in chapters 23 and 24. For now,
let's just get an idea of what disorientation is, and
what it feels like.

Disorientation is a common occurrence. With very
few exceptions, it happens to everyone at times.
Disorientation is the natural function of a normal brain.
It occurs when we are overwhelmed by stimuli or
thought. It also occurs when the brain receives conflicting
information from the different senses and attempts to
correlate the information.

15

A Clue About Disorientation

During my first year of college, I got a bad cold that developed into a severe inner-ear infection. I lay delirious in the hospital for two days, then woke up experiencing uncontrollable disorientation. Sounds were so loud they were painful to hear. I saw multiple images. My fingers wouldn't do what I wanted them to do. When I opened my eyes, all my senses told me I was spinning in space.

When I asked the doctor what was happening, he told me that it was because my brain was receiving and sending conflicting sensory perceptions.

"Your inner ears have two organs that tell your brain which way is up," he explained. "The right one is working, but the left one is telling your brain that *up* is some other direction. The two signals don't agree, so you feel like you're spinning around.

"But I can see that I'm spinning," I said. "Why is that?"

"Your senses aren't allowed to disagree," said the doctor. "It seems to be the way the brain is constructed. Your vision is adjusting to make the signals agree with each other. The spinning you see is tracking with the distortions in your sense of balance."

At the time, it helped to know that what I was experiencing was a result of the illness, and that the distortions would go away. Later on, when I began researching disorientation, this clue stuck in my mind. It explained why a distortion of one perception causes the others to shift correspondingly.

If you stand up and spin around quickly ten times, you will experience disorientation in the form of dizziness. If you stare at a spinning disk with a spiral painted on it, you will experience disorientation in the form of perceived movement. If you sit in your car at a stop sign and the car ahead of you rolls backward, you are likely to get the physical sensation that your own car is moving forward and press harder on the brake before you even think about it.

During a disorientation, your brain sees things moving that really aren't, or your body feels as if you are moving when you really aren't. Your sense of time can slow down or speed up. Your brain alters your actual perceptions, and you experience the altered perceptions as reality.

Whenever disorientation occurs, all the senses (except the sense of taste) are altered. The brain no longer sees what the eyes are seeing, but an altered perception of the images. The brain no longer hears what the ears are hearing, but an altered perception of the sounds. And so on through the rest of the perceptions, including the senses of touch, balance, motion and time.

The Dyslexic Dilemma

While disorientation is a common experience, dyslexics have taken it far beyond the ordinary. They don't just experience disorientation, they cause it to occur without realizing it.

Dyslexics use disorientation on an unconscious level

17

in order to perceive multidimensionally. By shifting their senses, they are able to experience multiple views of the world. They can perceive things from more than one perspective and gain more information from these perceptions than other people.

Apparently, as infants they somehow found a way to access the disorientation function of the brain and incorporated it into their thought and recognition processes. For infants who can't easily move around to examine things, being able to "fill in the blanks" and see things mentally from more than one perspective comes in handy.

Because the altered perceptions bring about recognition of objects that would otherwise be unrecognizable, disorientation becomes a normal part of dyslexics' thinking process. They are not aware of what occurs during the disorientation because it happens too fast. They are only aware of what occurs when they use it: better recognition of three-dimensional objects, sounds and tactile stimuli. Besides resolving confusion, dyslexics utilize the altered perceptions that occur with disorientations for creative imagination. When it is applied to solving a problem during nonverbal conceptualization, it might be called intuition, invention or inspiration. When it is done for entertainment, it is called fantasizing or daydreaming.

More about the inherent *talents* of dyslexics will be covered later. For now, it is enough to say that incorporating disorientation into the thought process can make dyslexics more perceptive or imaginative than the average person. When they begin to use language, it also creates the potential for developing a learning disability.

Until now, the dyslexic has been using disorientation to *resolve* confusion. This worked fine when dealing with real physical objects, so the dyslexic is likely to unconsciously disorient when a confusing symbol is encountered. Unfortunately, viewing a printed word on a page from the top or the back side, or scrambled into its component parts, makes the word more confusing than ever.

While learning to read, as confusions pile up, dyslexics will quickly reach their threshold of confusion. At this point, the dyslexic is no longer seeing what is actually written on the page, but what he or she *thinks* is on the page. Because the symbol isn't an object, and represents only the sound of a word that describes an object, action or idea, disorientation won't aid in its recognition. Because the symbol isn't recognized, the dyslexic will make a mistake. These mistakes are the primary symptoms of dyslexia.

CHAPTER 4

Dyslexia in Action

There are more than 200 English words that cause problems for most dyslexics. They are in the dyslexic's speaking vocabulary, but the dyslexic cannot form mental pictures of their meanings. That means the average dyslexic uses more than 200 words in speech that he or she cannot really think with. These little words—seemingly the most simple words in the language—are the stimuli or triggers for the symptoms of dyslexia.

Trigger words have abstract meanings, and often a number of different meanings. They trip up dyslexics because they do not represent visual objects or actions. They also happen to be the words that occur most frequently in everyday speech and writing. A complete list of trigger words is in chapter 35.

Origin of the Trigger Word List

I didn't invent this list. Like so many other discoveries related to my work, it came with a degree of surprise and the thought, "It's so obvious, I should have known it all along."

Soon after I made my initial discovery about perception, it became apparent to me that confusion triggered disorientations, and that confusion occurred whenever the person did not recognize a symbol. I thought each dyslexic would have a small, unique list of trigger words. Our programs included teaching students to notice disorientations when they occurred and to compile a list of their trigger words, so they would know which words to master.

As I made my own list, I was surprised. It wasn't at all what I thought it would be. I was embarrassed that it contained both of the one-letter words, all the two-letter words, and mostly four-letter words. I felt better when our clients listed the same words, but I still wondered why.

One evening in August 1982, I was looking over the Dolch List of basic sight words used by elementary teachers. I checked off a few words and pondered why some (such as *a*, *and* and *the*) triggered disorientations, and others (such as *home*, *food* and *friend*) didn't trigger dyslexic symptoms. I began to carefully examine my mental processes as I read each word. Like in a cartoon where the lightbulb goes on above a head, my realization lit up my universe. I discovered that I had no mental pictures for the trigger words. I couldn't picture them, so I couldn't think with them.

From the Dolch List I was able to identify 196 words that trigger disorientation. Today, the list has grown to 217 words. Most of the additions are contractions or other forms of words from the original list.

How Trigger Words Cause Problems

To put the puzzle pieces together, let's look at a typical scenario of a dyslexic child trying to read aloud.

A simple sentence like the one below would be easy to read for a ten-year-old who thinks with the sounds of words. But for a ten-year-old dyslexic who constructs mental pictures of the scene as each word is read, the process is more difficult.

> *The brown horse jumped over the stone fence and ran through the pasture.*

For the ten-year-old dyslexic, the first word, *The*, caused the mental imagery to go blank, because there was no picture for it. A blank picture is the essence of confusion; nothing a person experiences can match the confusion it causes. Using concentration, however, the child pushes past the blank picture and says "the," and forces himself to skip to the next word.

The word *brown* produces a mental image of a color, but it has no defined shape. Continuing to concentrate, he says "brown."

The word *horse* transforms the brown picture into a horse of that color. Concentration continues and "horse" is said.

The word *jumped* causes the front of the brown horse to rise into the air. He continues concentrating as he says "jumped."

The word *over* causes the back of the brown horse to rise. Still concentrating, he says "over."

The next word, another *the*, causes the picture to go blank again. Confusion for the reader has increased, but the threshold of confusion has not yet been reached. He must now double his concentration so he can push on to the next word. In doing so, he may or may not omit saying "the."

The word *stone* produces a picture of a rock. With concentration doubled, he says "stone."

The next word, *fence*, turns the rock into a rock fence. Still with doubled concentration, he says "fence."

The next word, *and*, blanks out the picture again. This time, the threshold for confusion is reached. So the child becomes disoriented. The child is stopped again, more confused, doubly concentrating, and now disoriented. The only way he can continue is to increase his concentration effort. But now because he is also disoriented, the dyslexic symptoms will appear. It is very likely that he will omit saying the word *and*, or just as likely that he will substitute *a*, *an* or *the* instead. At this point, he is no longer getting an accurate perception of the words on the page.

He is now expending a tremendous amount of effort and energy on concentrating, just to continue.

The next word, *ran*, because he is now disoriented, is altered into the word *runs*. He sees an image of himself running, entirely unrelated to the picture of the hovering horse. Then he says "runs."

The word *through* is altered into *throws*. He sees himself throwing a ball and says "throws."

The next word, *the*, blanks out the picture again. The child is stopped again, even more confused, and still disoriented. His only recourse is to quadruple his concentration. In doing so, he omits saying "the."

By now his disorientation has created a feeling like dizziness. He is feeling sick to his stomach, and the words and letters are swimming around on the page.

For the last word, *pasture*, he must track down each letter, one at a time, so he can sound out the word. Once he does, he sees a picture of a grassy place. Even though he is disoriented, because of the extra effort and energy he put forth in catching and sounding out each letter, he says it right, "pasture."

Having completed the sentence, he closes the book and pushes it away. That's enough of that!

When asked what he just read, he is likely to answer with something like "a place where grass grows." He has a picture of a horse in the air, a stone fence, himself playing ball and a grassy place, but cannot relate the separate elements in the sentence to form a mental image of the scene described.

To everyone who saw or heard him read the sentence or heard his answer to what it was about, it's obvious that he didn't understand any of what he just read. As for him, he doesn't care that he didn't understand it. He's just thankful that he survived the ordeal of reading out loud.

Word	Reaction	Sees/Thinks	Says
The	picturing process stops; concentration begins	blank picture	*the*
brown	concentration continues	brown color	*brown*
horse	concentration continues	brown horse	*horse*
jumped	concentration continues	front of the horse rises	*jumped*
over	concentration continues	back of horse rises	*over*
the	picturing process stops; concentration doubles	blank picture	*the*
stone	doubled concentration	a rock	*stone*
fence	doubled concentration	rock fence	*fence*
and	picturing process stops; disorientation occurs; concentration triples	blank picture	*(omits word?)*
ran	disorientation continues; tripled concentration	running	*runs*
through	disorientation continues; tripled concentration	throwing a ball	*throws*
the	picturing process stops; disorientation continues; concentration quadruples	blank picture	*(omits word)*
pasture	disorientation continues; quadrupled concentration	a grassy place	*pasture*

If he were a little older he would realize that he just read something that he didn't understand. So what would he probably do? *Read it again.* It seems logical that if we read it again we'll get more out of it—doesn't it? Look again at the scenario above and ask the question, "What has changed that will make reading the sentence any different the second time?" *Nothing!*

When reading important or technical data, adult dyslexics will reread the material between three and ten times before they feel they understand it, or they will abandon the attempt.

Isn't Concentration Good?

I should clarify a point here about concentration: Most people consider it a positive ability, but too much of anything, even something positive, can be detrimental. The degree to which the dyslexic must concentrate to push past a blank picture definitely produces a negative effect.

When people concentrate on something, they are putting most of their awareness on that thing. When they are intensely concentrating, they are *limiting* their awareness to *only* that thing.

This is a fundamental aspect of hypnotism. It is the exact mechanism used by hypnotists to put someone into a trance. When dyslexics intensely concentrate in order to read, they experience a hypnotic state that adds to the difficulty of understanding the material read, as well as the time required to comprehend it.

CHAPTER 5

Compulsive Solutions

Once disorientations begin to cause mistakes, the dyslexic child becomes frustrated. Nobody likes to make mistakes, so around the age of nine, in about third grade, the dyslexic child begins to find, figure out and adopt solutions to the problem. Even though this may seem like a good thing, it is actually how the reading problem becomes a true learning disability.

The solutions dyslexics invent don't solve the real problem of distorted perceptions; they only afford temporary relief from frustrations. They are roundabout methods of coping with the effects of disorientation. They ultimately slow down the learning process and form the real learning disability.

These "solutions" are methods of doing things and tactics for knowing or remembering things. They quickly become compulsive behaviors. Once a dyslexic adopts one, it will be the only way he can perform that particular function. During the process of correcting dyslexia, I refer to them as "old solutions," because they are no longer needed.

Although many dyslexics begin developing compulsive solutions before the age of nine, and continue to develop more for the rest of their lives, most of these "learning crutches" are developed between the ages of nine and twelve. Dyslexics usually have hundreds if not thousands of them.

Here are a few common examples of compulsive solutions.

The Alphabet Song

A common childhood solution is reciting the "Alphabet Song." If the song is learned at home or in kindergarten as a simple training pattern, within two years most children will be able to recite the alphabet without either singing the song or replaying it mentally. But if children adopt the song as a solution to not being able to learn the alphabet, they will never be able to recite the alphabet without either singing it out loud or replaying it mentally.

They know only the song; the song knows the alphabet. So by using the song, they can *appear* to know the alphabet. Whenever they want to look up a name in the phone book or a word in the dictionary, the song will be used. It has become a compulsive behavior.

Heavy Concentration

Of all the compulsive solutions dyslexics come up with, probably the worst one is "concentration." Before learning how to concentrate, most dyslexics can't read at all. Once they learn to concentrate hard enough, they do learn how to read—slowly and laboriously. The problem is that reading will be unpleasant and painful for them. If what they are trying to read is important, they will have to read it over and over many times to make sure it's correct. They won't read for pleasure, because there is no pleasure in heavy concentration.

Probably the most common characteristics of dyslexia in adults are slow reading, going over the same material many times and tension headaches caused by the heavy concentration they use to read.

There is a clear distinction with dyslexics between concentration and *paying attention.* Paying attention to something interesting is fun. Concentration on something life-threatening is no fun at all. In fact, it is highly stressful. The inability to read and write often seems life-threatening to a dyslexic person.

"Do It for Me"

For adult dyslexics, an easier solution than heavy concentration is getting other people to read and write things for them. You may have been tricked into doing this by someone who said, "Would you read this and tell me what you think of it?"

Do you remember how that person fished for more information? It was a ploy, even though you probably didn't notice. Your opinion really wasn't what they were after; it was the information contained in whatever you were asked to read. Your reading skills were utilized by a dyslexic who couldn't decipher the words on the page and got you to interpret them.

Some brilliant dyslexics become corporate executives because of their intuitive gifts for "seeing" the correct strategy and mobilizing the work force. They will always invest heavily in the latest dictation and video equipment—anything that transmits information in a form other than writing. They will rely on trusted subordinates to read things for them and relay messages that must be delivered in writing. That's because they are secretly functional illiterates.

For Better or for Worse?

It is ironic that many of the "best" teaching and tutoring techniques used to help dyslexics do nothing more than implant and reinforce compulsive behaviors. This is understandable, because it appears the dyslexic is finally beginning to learn.

This is only an illusion. The child is actually being

conditioned into performing rote acts that aren't really understood. This conditioning will be a lifetime disability unless it is corrected at some point in the future.

CHAPTER 6

Problems with Reading

(Especially English)

You may have forgotten what it was like to learn to read. Most people who can read fairly well do it automatically, unaware of how many gyrations their minds are going through. Reading is considered by many researchers to be the most complex function we require our brains to perform.

Maybe you have heard about computer software that performs optical character recognition. It "reads" an image of print and converts it into text characters that can be used in a computer program. The Postal Service uses it to read typed ZIP codes for mail sorting. These programs take some time and require considerable processing to work as they crawl along, letter by letter. They also tend to make many mistakes. It's a wonder they work at all, considering the complexity of what they have to do.

When you read, your brain has to do the same thing

(though you probably recognize many entire words). Then you have to look up the words in your mental dictionary and string them together so they make sense within the context of a complete sentence or thought. You are actually converting characters into word sounds, then combining those words into speech. For a dyslexic, this poses two problems.

First, when disoriented, a dyslexic's optical character recognition software isn't getting a clear picture of the characters on the page—it's trying to read the equivalent of a poor copy, so it makes more mistakes.

Secondly, dyslexics don't really "hear" thoughts internally. This means they don't mentally sound out the words as they read. In fact, despite the current popularity of phonic methods to teach reading, dyslexics usually do better at sight reading, where they simply recognize an individual word as a concept.

The problems dyslexics have in learning to read are the same as those all children experience, but of a larger magnitude. They are made worse by inconsistencies in the language. If the printed word were presented more consistently, especially in beginning schoolbooks, some of these problems would be lessened for all children.

The Problem with Typography

Until the early twentieth century, all printing looked pretty similar. This was because when text was prepared for printing, typographers used characters made from individual metal castings. A printer could afford only so many sets of type, and they had to fit together uniformly in a row. The main exception was hand-painted signs and posters.

Today, thanks to computerized typesetting, we have a wealth of styles to choose from. Graphic designers can express themselves even further by warping, bending and otherwise distorting type styles. This makes the printed page look more artistic but less legible, especially to dyslexics who are adding distortions of their own every time they come across a word or symbol that causes them to disorient.

This is true even of dictionaries used by schoolchildren. For example, here are the beginnings of three entries from a "young people's" dictionary. What do you think they say?

III
I'll
Ill.

Here are the complete entries:

III a Roman numeral for the figure 3.
I'll 1. I shall. 2. I will.
Ill. abbreviation for Illinois.

Note that you cannot really tell whether the abbreviation for Illinois is the Roman numeral three, since either one would normally be followed by a period. Nor is there any way to tell the capital *I* from the lowercase *L*.

Here are a few examples of different type styles. As an experiment, try turning this book upside down or hold it in front of a mirror and see which ones are harder to read. You'll probably find those that give you the most trouble are the most unusual ones, or those with the most complex decorative elements. Those are the typefaces that tend to give dyslexics the most trouble.

ABCDEFGHIJKLMNOPQRSTUVWXYZ
zyxwvutsrqponmlkjihgfedcba   *1234567890*

ABCDEFGHIJKLMNOPQRSTUVWXYZ
ZYXWVUTSRQPONMLKJIHGFEDCBA   **1234567890**

ABCDEFGHIJKLMNOPQRSTUVWXYZ
zyxwvutsrqponmlkjihgfedcba   1234567890

ABCDEFGHIJKLMNOPQRSTUVWXYZ
ZYXWVUTSRQPONMLKJIHGFEDCBA   **1234567890**

𝔄𝔅ℭ𝔇𝔈𝔉𝔊ℌℑ𝔍𝔎𝔏𝔐𝔑𝔒𝔓𝔔ℜ𝔖𝔗𝔘𝔙𝔚𝔛𝔜ℨ
zyxwvutsrqponmlkjihgfedcba   1234567890

ABCDEFGHIJKLMNOPQRSTUVWXYZ
zyxwvutsrqponmlkjihgfedcba   **1234567890**

ABCDEFGHIJKLMNOPQRSTUVWXYZ
zyxwvutsrqponmlkjihgfedcba   *1234567890*

ABCDEFGHIJKLMNOPQRSTUVWXYZ
zyxwvutsrqponmlkjihgfedcba   1234567890

ABCDEFGHIJKLMNOPQRSTUVWXYZ
zyxwvutsrqponmlkjihgfedcba   1234567890

ABCDEFGHIJKLMNOPQRSTUVWXYZ
zyxwvutsrqponmlkjihgfedcba 1234567890

Alphabetical Obstacles

Our alphabet is not phonetically accurate. In order to represent all the possible sounds of speech, it would need about 44 characters. The Russian alphabet, for instance, has 32 characters, not 26. Some languages have 50 characters or more. This eliminates the need for some characters or combinations of characters to represent as many as five different sounds as they do in English. If you read aloud in some languages and simply pronounce the letters phonetically, you will say every word correctly without guessing about the sounds you are supposed to make.

Even other languages that use the same characters as English, such as Spanish, French and Portuguese, make liberal use of accents over certain letters, like *a* and *e*, to help people pronounce them accurately. The Spanish are polite enough to warn us beforehand that a sentence is going to be a question by putting an upside-down question mark at the beginning.

Naturally, dyslexia is a worldwide phenomenon, at least in places where written languages are made up of sound symbols. The variations in cultures and teaching methods would make it difficult to discern the exact influence of different languages on the learning process. But common sense tells me that English, with its multitude of inconsistencies, is one of the more difficult languages for dyslexics to pronounce and spell correctly.

It might help if teachers explained to students that our language is a rather messy system, with so many variations and exceptions to the rules that the rules often don't work at all.

Reading is not the only place where dyslexia symptoms show up. Because dyslexics naturally respond to confusion by becoming disoriented, wherever we find symbols—spoken or written—we can find symptoms. The other most common areas are spelling, math, and handwriting. Symptons are also common with attention deficits and hyperactivity.

CHAPTER 7

Spelling Problems

The spelling problems dyslexics have are mostly the result of disorientation. When a disorientation occurs, the person gets multiple views of the word. Not only is it looked at forward, backward and upside down both ways, it is pulled apart and reassembled in every possible combination. There are at least 40 different variations of a three-letter word such as "cat," and only six of these are "logical" versions, with the letters in their correct configurations (see illustration on page 86).

These variations, of course, only involve rearranging the letters two-dimensionally. Dyslexics often see the letters three-dimensionally, as if they were floating in space. This creates an infinite number of different views. One little girl said the letters crawled off the page and hid in the carpet.

The Rules Don't Work

Teaching a person spelling rules is frustrating, because there are so many exceptions to the rules. One out of six words is phonetically irregular. If you teach a corrected dyslexic the rules, his spelling scores may actually go down. This is because when spelling is tested, it is usually to see whether the person knows the exceptions to the rules. If he follows the rules strictly, the test will be a disaster.

Once perception is accurate, spelling improvement will follow. Symbol Mastery (chapters 33 and 35) and Spell-Reading (chapter 34) are the best methods I have discovered to teach dyslexics to recognize and spell words they will need to use in everyday reading and writing.

A written word is nothing more than a symbol composed of one or more alphabet symbols. The symbols together indicate what it looks like (on paper), what it sounds like (when someone says it) and what it means. Spelling is only the "what it looks like" component. When the word is mastered using Symbol Mastery, the person learns all three parts, and can utilize the word fully in reading, speaking and thinking.

How Important Is It?

Our educational system has an obsession with spelling-bee correctness. It wasn't always so. In Elizabethan

England, many variations were acceptable as long as people could figure out how the word was supposed to sound. Spelling styles have changed considerably over the years, as you can tell by looking at a replica of the original U.S. Declaration of Independence. How do you think Thomas Jefferson would do in a spelling bee today?

Instead of turning spelling into a contest, it's better to simply point out the difference between the word the student wrote and the correct spelling (or spellings) in the dictionary. Eventually, corrected dyslexics will figure out on their own how to spell the words as they read. As improvement occurs, it is important not to criticize students or make them feel wrong for making errors.

If a student continues to make spelling mistakes by attempting to spell words phonetically, blame it on our imprecise system of phonetics, not on the student.

CHAPTER 8

Math Problems

Not all dyslexics have problems with math. When they do, it is usually called *acalculia* or *dyscalculia.* Many common difficulties with math result from the methods that are used in attempting to teach it. But the dyslexic has an underlying problem that can make learning math difficult, if not impossible.

Acalculia and dyscalculia can be traced directly to the time-sense distortions that are common among dyslexic children. They occur simultaneously with visual, auditory and balance/motion disorientations.

The Mental Time Clock

Everyone experiences time-sense distortion to some degree. It is usually related to the emotions of boredom and excitement. When you become bored, your internal clock speeds up, and time seems to drag. When you become excited, your internal clock slows down and time seems to fly by. These distortions are minor compared to those a dyslexic experiences during periods of disorientation. If the dyslexic is a dancer, athlete or firefighter, the ability to experience time in slow motion can be a great advantage. This is why some dancers and basketball players are able to give the appearance of "hovering in midair."

I theorize that, biochemically, a person's time sense is primarily controlled by the amount of the neurotransmitter dopamine around the synapses of the brain. The more dopamine, the faster the internal clock goes. The faster it goes, the more external time seems to slow down. The less dopamine, the slower the clock goes. External time seems to speed up. Disorientations seem to cause a change in the amount of dopamine that is created and dispersed in the brain.

Disorientation is a constant mental companion to dyslexic children. As they go through childhood, distorted perception is as common as actual perception. Because of this, most dyslexic children have little sense of time. Ordinary children experience time rather consistently. By the age of seven, they can estimate the passage of time with fair accuracy. For the dyslexic, time has never been consistently experienced, so estimating its passage may be impossible.

Without an inherent sense of time, understanding the concept of *sequence*—the way things follow each other, one after another—would be difficult if not impossible. Even simple counting is a matter of sequence. So the seven-year-old dyslexic also could lack this inherent concept.

Without the concepts of time and sequence, an accurate understanding of the concept of "order versus disorder" is doubtful.

The Basics of Math

All math, from simple arithmetic to astrophysics calculus, is composed of order (versus disorder), sequence and time. Children who have an inherent sense of these three concepts can learn and understand math. For children who do not possess these concepts, learning math is reduced to memorization. The extent to which they will be able to use math is limited by their ability to remember the rote procedures. Without an understanding of these underlying concepts, there will never be any real understanding of the subject or its principles.

For a dyslexic to learn math, these basics must be mastered:

1. *Time*, meaning the measurement of change in relation to a standard.
2. *Sequence*, meaning the way things follow each other, one after another in amount, in size, in time, in arbitrary (man-made) order or in importance.

3. *Order*, meaning things in their proper places, proper positions and proper conditions.

Once these concepts are mastered, accurate counting can be mastered. Then learning arithmetic may change from a labor to a joy.

An interesting side note is that mathematics and music are composed of the same three elements: order, sequence and time. They are just expressed in different mediums. So it shouldn't be surprising that many top mathematicians are also excellent musicians, and vice versa.

CHAPTER 9

Handwriting Problems

When a dyslexic has a writing problem, it is usually diagnosed as *agraphia* or *dysgraphia.* It is related to disorientation. There are several reasons for writing problems. Sometimes poor writing is used to cover up spelling problems or other deficiencies. Sometimes it is simply because writing instructions were given while the dyslexic was disoriented.

Multiple Mental Pictures

The most common type of writing problem occurs when dyslexic students have had so much instruction on what their writing *should* look like that they have multiple mental pictures of words and letters superimposed over one another. With a pen or pencil they can make only one line at a time, so what they draw is a combination of all of these pictures, usually switching from one to another. The result is a jumble of lines that wiggle and jump all over the paper.

The solution is to get rid of all the old mental pictures. Once the pictures are gone, the person can see a clear, single mental picture of what writing should look like. In these cases, it is fortunate that dyslexics have such vivid mental images. By following the simple procedure of having the person access and erase the superfluous pictures one by one, it is easy to eliminate them.

Dormant Neural Pathways

The worst type of writing problem is the most difficult to explain because of the biophysics of how the brain processes stimuli and produces function.

Picture the brain as a large fishing net. There are vertical cords and horizontal cords, and every place the cords cross there is a knot. In this model, the cords would be neurons and the knots would be synapses. By tracing along the cords, you can move from any knot to any other knot in the net. So theoretically every synapse of the brain is connected to every other synapse.

Add to the picture that the net is divided into several hundred different areas, and each area provides a different service to the whole. There are seeing areas, hearing areas, finger-wiggling areas and so on for everything humans can perceive and do.

As a perceptual stimulus comes into the net, the first knot is stimulated. From there the signal is processed by sending other stimuli along other cords to other knots, and so on, until the original stimulus has reached all the knots it must reach. There are an untold number of different paths this stimulus could follow, but once a particular path is used, it becomes stronger. The stronger it is, the more it is used. Also, there are certain paths that never get stimulated, so they remain weak and unused.

Consider that the paths are neural pathways, and that as a unit they form a neural network. Now consider that because of a dyslexic's distorted perceptions (disorientation), the neural pathway for seeing straight diagonal lines has never been stimulated. This person would simply not be able to see straight diagonal lines.

This isn't to say the person's eyes wouldn't pass along the images correctly. The problem is that the brain wouldn't process diagonal line images. The neural pathways for processing the stimuli have never been used. Also, because the brain has never been able to see a straight diagonal line, it cannot instruct the hand to draw one, because the neural pathway for making one has never been used.

Because a dysgraphic child needs to make straight diagonal lines in writing, but has never seen one, the child will draw what he or she saw. The distorted perception that was formed when looking at straight diagonal lines will be the model for what the "make the line" neural pathway will tell the hand to produce.

This is a simplistic model, but the principle is accurate. I have worked with many dyslexics who simply couldn't see diagonal lines. Using clay, they could not form letters with diagonal lines such as *A, M, N, W, V* and *X*. Usually *W* is the worst. These people just can't figure out how to attach four straight ropes of clay together to make them look like a *W.*

Sometimes when moms or teachers are watching me work with such a person, they become frustrated because the student can't seem to make it happen. I don't get frustrated, because I know what is really happening.

Once the person is oriented, I know that the neural pathways for seeing straight diagonal lines can now be stimulated. They are no longer blocked because of distortions. I also know that the person is opening up previously unused neural pathways at each attempt to put the pieces of clay together. It doesn't take long, usually less than an hour, before the pathway is opened and the person creates a diagonal line. Once the pathway opens, it becomes stronger and stronger. Usually within a day or two, the person can see all the straight diagonal lines in the surrounding environment that have been invisible or distorted up to that point.

In the example, I used straight diagonal lines. In real life it is not limited to that. The same thing can happen with any number of visual stimuli. It is remedied by providing stimuli to the person in a correctly oriented condition, then having him create the missing information using Symbol Mastery.

May 14

"See what I DID?" (Sade) Andy.
I ash you! , is that a drawing
you Bo n't is (Sade) Bety
when. see saw it.
Yes, it is (Sade) joe,
It has a lot in it
come on

May 16

Agenst the darkgrownd I can tell
you the absolutly the best
flirt I ever made never left
inside a brick bilding at
Kennedy Airport Airport
It was in TWA's 747 simulator.

May 17

I'm going to go all over. First I'm
going to Saint Louis for my family
reunion on my mom's side. Then I'm
going to a neat camp up in Mendocino
called Camp Winarainbow. After that
I might go to Idaho to visit my
uncle.

*Handwriting samples made by an eleven-year-old boy with agraphia
during the Davis Dyslexia Correction Program.*

"How Did You Do That?"

We're often asked how the changes in handwriting illustrated on the previous page could have occurred in only four days.

This boy had a genius IQ. At age eleven, he was reading the encyclopedia for pleasure, and dictating full-length plays and short novels to his mother. Each time he tried to write, however, he would break the pencil lead after only a few words. His primary goal was to overcome his agraphia and learn to write cursive.

The underlying cause of his agraphia was a combination of strong disorientations in the senses of vision and motion, multiple mental pictures of what written words *should* look like and undeveloped neural pathways for seeing certain types or attitudes of lines.

The first step in correcting his agraphia was Orientation Counseling. Then he completed Alphabet and Punctuation Marks Mastery as described in chapter 33.

Another step in addressing his handwriting problem was to give him a sample of each letter and ask him to copy it. Those he could not write required motions that triggered disorientations. Once these were located, each motion was practiced one at a time, first in space and then very large on paper, until they no longer triggered disorientations. These included many of the loops and changes in direction used in cursive writing.

His pencil grip was addressed by having him practice large drawing motions with a marker on a large piece of paper. The size was gradually decreased until he could use a pencil or pen on a piece of paper to make small marks and doodles.

Finally he practiced writing a word. After each attempt, he was asked if he had any mental pictures of what that word *should* look like and told to erase all the pictures. This was repeated until he no longer had a picture of what the word "should" look like and had only a single picture. This procedure was repeated with many words, to a point where he spontaneously erased all his past pictures of "what words should look like." At that point, with simple penmanship instruction, he quickly learned to write.

CHAPTER 10

Attention Focus:
ADD and ADHD

The main thing new about *attention deficit disorder*, or ADD, is the use of these words to describe a learning disability. The problem has been around ever since teachers have attempted to teach students subjects that didn't interest them. In most cases, it should be described not as a learning disability, but as a teaching disability.

There is a genuine medical disorder called ADD that prevents a person from maintaining attention. It would certainly hinder performance in school if it were the real problem. For parents whose child is being forced to take medications, I recommend a trip to the library. Look up the condition in *The Merck Manual* or *DSM-IV*, the standard diagnostic guides used by physicians. See whether it actually describes your child.

Currently, many students who cannot maintain fixed attention on a task for very long are being diagnosed as suffering from ADD. They are said to be "easily distractible." They shift their attention to other things in the environment instead of sticking to what the teacher has assigned.

Sometimes the ADD problem is accompanied by a second condition called hyperactivity. Both are rooted in the developmental differences of dyslexic children during early childhood.

Different Learning Styles

"Normal" children bring to the classroom an underlying characteristic that dyslexic children lack. A child who isn't dyslexic has already begun to develop the ability to concentrate prior to starting school. A dyslexic child probably won't begin developing this questionable ability until about the age of nine, or about third grade.

Dyslexic children can access and use their mental function of distorted perception to bring about recognition of objects and events in the environment. This is their natural, normal reaction to the feeling of confusion. When they use the distorted perception function, they achieve recognition and the feeling of confusion disappears. Because of this, most dyslexic children aren't well accustomed to the feeling of confusion. When it happens, it is almost instantly eliminated.

Other preschoolers go through periods of prolonged confusion, if for no other reason than their inability to eliminate it.

The feeling of confusion draws more and more attention to the source of the confusion. The end result of prolonged confusion is concentration, simply because most of the child's attention is being fixed upon whatever caused the confusion. Children who do not have a method of quickly eliminating confusion develop the ability to concentrate. Dyslexic children do not develop this ability at an early age because the stimuli for developing it can be eliminated so quickly and easily.

Attention vs. Concentration

It is natural and easy for dyslexic children to pay attention, but difficult for them to concentrate. There is a tremendous difference between the two. When people are paying attention, their awareness is spread out; it can encompass the entire immediate environment. When people are concentrating, all or most or their attention is fixed on only one thing in the immediate environment.

My opinion is that heavy concentration produces a superficial, rote type of learning, characterized by memorization without full understanding. Children who learn in this way can go through the motions, but don't fully get the underlying concepts of the subjects being taught.

While watching TV or playing with toys, the more interested or curious a child is in the experience, the more attention the child will put on it. But there is still some attention left over for the rest of the environment. In other words, the child is paying more attention to one thing, but is still not abandoning or excluding the rest of the environment. This is true of ordinary children as well as dyslexics, but the dyslexic child will keep attention more widely spread around the environment than the ordinary child.

Curiosity

Because dyslexic children are generally so environ-mentally aware, they tend to be curious. Curiosity, more than anything else, can cause them to shift their attention. If they find the object of curiosity interesting, they will pay more attention to it than to other things in the environment. They automatically put most of their attention on whatever they find most interesting.

If a dyslexic child sitting in a classroom hears a noise outside, or something moves past the window, or a student in the next row drops something, instantly the dyslexic's attention shifts to the distraction. The other students and possibly the teacher weren't even aware anything happened. But the dyslexic student naturally reacted because he or she noticed it and became curious about what it might be.

Boredom also plays a role, because boredom often happens to someone whose mind is working between 400 and 2,000 times faster than the minds of the people around them. A dyslexic child who is bored will do one of two things. Either the child will disorient into creative imagination (daydreaming), or will shift his attention to something that *is* interesting (distractibility or inattention).

The impulsive aspect of ADD is most prevalent when the student is confused or uncertain about what to do. Otherwise, it is usually just an attempt to overcome agonizing boredom.

There is a growing recognition that the symptoms of ADD, like those of dyslexia, can be an advantage in many real-life situations. The potential benefits have been explored in a number of books on the subject. Some of these are listed in the Recommended References section at the end of this book.

A highly regimented classroom is not a real-life situation by any stretch of the imagination.

If a teacher does not appeal to the curiosity of a student and has failed to make the subject being taught the most interesting thing in the environment, the teacher has created the perfect environment for ADD. This teacher will eventually tell the parents of a dyslexic child that the child can't stay on task, is easily distractible and should be tested.

Hyperactivity

When ADD is accompanied by hyperactivity, it creates a bigger problem in the classroom, so the child is more likely to be singled out for diagnosis and treatment, often with Ritalin, Adderall, Strattera or other drugs. Hyperactivity is simply the addition of physical movement by the student.

Dyslexic children often get tagged with the *hyper* label because of the physical effects of disorientation. Most students simply become bored and struggle to stay awake when they are disinterested or confused. Dyslexics also become disoriented.

The mechanism of hyperactivity is easy to understand when viewed from the following perspective. First the student isn't interested in what is going on, and doesn't understand what the teacher is saying. The resulting boredom and confusion activate the perception-altering function of the brain, and the student becomes disoriented. While bored, confused and therefore disoriented, the student's internal clock speeds up, so perceived external time seems to slow down. For every minute of actual time, this student must endure two minutes of trying to stay out of trouble, pay attention, concentrate or sit still.

The student's senses are distorted, including the senses of balance and movement. The senses of balance and movement register in only two ways. Either you are still or moving; either you are balanced or out of balance. If the student is sitting still when the distortions begin, he or she will have the sense of moving. If the student sits still long enough, motion sickness will set in. If the student begins to move, the sensations will reverse and the student will feel as if he or she is sitting still. This is why the student begins to move around: to compensate for the feeling of motion sickness and keep from having an upset stomach or throwing up. This may be why Ritalin, a stimulant, works in reverse and seems to slow down "hyperactive" grade-schoolers.

Because the student's perceptions are distorted and the offensive movement is a product of these distorted perceptions, every time he or she is told to *sit still*, the movement will increase. This happens because the senses of balance and movement are reversed. If the student learned how to achieve orientation, the perception distortion function of the brain could be turned off. The student could perceive the environment accurately. The need to move to compensate for the distorted balance and movement perceptions would be gone.

Learning to become oriented stops the disorientation symptoms, but it will never make a student interested in a subject that is poorly taught. It is interesting that very good teachers rarely seem to have students with ADD in their classes, even though some of the same students are labeled as suffering from ADD in other classes.

CHAPTER 11

Clumsiness

Some dyslexics suffer from a particular type of chronic clumsiness called dyspraxia. It isn't always associated with dyslexia because it doesn't directly affect reading, writing, spelling or math. It is most commonly considered an auditory deficit.

It's likely that the phrase "He can't walk and chew gum at the same time" was invented to describe a severely dyspraxic person. "Accident prone" is another common term for dyspraxia in our culture. One mother told me her son *never grew out of his awkward stage.*

Clumsiness isn't the only characteristic of dyspraxia. It is common that dyspraxic individuals will not look straight at you when they speak to you. Some will have a "wandering eye," where on occasion, one of their eyes drifts off and seems to be looking in a different direction. Often, when they read they hold the book crooked so they are reading up and down as opposed to side to side. If so, the same will occur when they write. The handwriting is almost always atrocious. When we consider distorted perception as the root of the problem, dyspraxia makes sense.

It appears that dyspraxia could have two causes. First, the sense of balance and movement could be distorted because of disorientation. This is obvious, because disorientation can cause the sensation of dizziness. However, distortion in perception can occur even when the person isn't disoriented. This is because the natural orientation isn't very good. Even when the perceptions stop distorting and become consistent for a while, they aren't accurate.

To better understand this, consider the two fundamental characteristics of optimum orientation: *consistent perception* and *accurate perception.* If we have consistent perception, even if it isn't accurate, we can learn how to read, write, spell and do math. Most non-dyslexic people have consistent perception because of their stable orientation, whereas dyslexics do not.

For all the senses except balance and motion, some degree of inaccuracy won't greatly affect the person's ability to read, listen, speak or write. A person who is tone-deaf won't be able to sing well, but can carry on a conversation with no trouble. A person who is color-blind won't be able to paint a realistic picture, but can easily read a newspaper article.

However, distortions in the senses of balance and motion will always cause some degree of clumsiness. The primary source of our senses of balance and motion are the *vestibular* organs in our inner ear. These organs have tiny "motion sensor" hairs in liquid-filled chambers that work on a similar principle to a carpenter's level. Imagine hanging some pictures on the wall with a level that is not aligned properly. You will end up with a wall full of consistently crooked pictures.

The senses of balance and motion are regulated by gravity and the environment. For uncorrected dyslexics with dyspraxia, even when they aren't disoriented, the natural orientation they experience is not providing them with accurate vestibular perception. Any distortion—even if it is consistent—will give the person an incorrect sense of the physical environment, and will become obvious in the person's physical responses.

Dyspraxia makes sense, because if the senses of balance and movement are either temporarily distorted or inherently inaccurate, we would expect to see clumsy or awkward behavior.

All dyslexics will, from time to time, experience some degree of dyspraxia because of disorientations. It shows up as a chronic condition in only about 10 to 15 percent of dyslexic children. Like the other aspects of dyslexia, it varies in severity.

The chronic clumsiness caused by inaccurate perception is solved when the Orientation and Fine

Tuning procedures are done. The sporadic clumsiness caused by disorientation will be gradually resolved as the dyslexia itself is solved by gaining mastery of the symbols of language. The auditory deficit aspect of dyspraxia will be resolved over time as the orientation becomes stable.

CHAPTER 12

A Real Solution

What every dyslexic needs is the ability to think with the symbols and words that trigger disorientation. These words are already part of the dyslexic's speaking vocabulary, but the dyslexic probably couldn't give a definition if asked for one, and doesn't have a mental picture of the word's meaning.

Until the person fully understands the trigger words and can use them in his or her thought process, any remedial work may make the problem worse, not better.

This seems to be a sticky situation. Dyslexics need to learn to think with the very words that cause disorientation. Being exposed to these words will cause them to distort the data they are trying to learn. If we provide a definition for the word, we have already defeated the purpose, because everything the dyslexic hears or reads in a disoriented state is altered and incorrect. It is like asking a person to walk into a fire without being burned.

The impasse is like a closed circuit or a catch-22. The action that should solve the problem is creating the problem.

Orientation Counseling

The way to move beyond this impasse is by giving the dyslexic a method to control the disorientations that occur when trigger words are encountered. There are two different procedures that can terminate a state of disorientation, called Orientation Counseling procedures: a simple technique called the Davis Alignment Procedure, which is a tactile/kinesthetic process, and the Davis Orientation Counseling Procedure, which is a visual process. Either procedure teaches the dyslexic a technique for terminating or turning off disorientations. Once the person learns how to eliminate the multiple perceptions, he can experience a consistent, undistorted viewpoint whenever he wishes. Once one of the techniques is learned, it will be simple to do anywhere, and will take less than a second to do. These counseling procedures are covered in chapters 27 and 30.

The result of *orientation* is an accurate, consistent perception of the environment, including two-dimensional words printed on a page. When the dyslexic is oriented, the words on the page are perceived correctly, without distortion. Data can be received accurately.

If a dyslexic can recognize disorientation and consciously produce a state of orientation at will, disorientation can be turned off whenever it occurs. Then the person can acquire the information he needs to learn. Even if disorienting stimuli are encountered and disorientation occurs, it can be corrected quickly. So it will no longer prevent accurate perception and learning.

The symptoms of dyslexia are manifestations of disorientation, so terminating the disorientation also terminates the symptoms. The reading skill of most dyslexics improves dramatically as soon as they begin to use this simple process. They may still have problems with words they don't know, but they are at least able to recognize the words they have already learned.

It may seem that the problem is solved simply by controlling the disorientations, but nothing has been done about the real problem at all. In fact, a new problem has been added: constantly checking one's state of orientation and making corrections to stop disorientation.

Symbol Mastery

Dyslexics need to learn to think nonverbally with trigger words. Once they do, there is no need to consciously control disorientations. It was the inability to think with the trigger words that caused the disorientations to occur in the first place. The ability to think with the trigger words will eliminate the disorientations.

This presents a new set of problems for educators. The traditional teaching methods used in the educational system—at least in the Western world—are not well suited to the thought process of a nonverbal thinker. Just having a dyslexic read the definitions of trigger words like *a, and* and *the* from the dictionary, even while maintaining orientation, will not allow the person to *think* with the words. The definitions are only being recited like the "Alphabet Song." The meanings of the words are not fully comprehended.

Dyslexics need to form mental pictures they can use to think with, and to associate these pictures visually and auditorily with the words they are trying to learn.

Showing a dyslexic a picture to describe the meaning of a word would seem to be a step in the right direction, but even that doesn't work very well. It requires a tremendous amount of repetition. You might have to flash a picture in front of a dyslexic a thousand times before the person could incorporate that picture into his or her thinking process. Dyslexics usually find rote repetition excruciatingly boring, so they are likely to disorient into their own thoughts and daydream rather than pay attention to this type of exercise.

Again, there seems to be an impasse. Traditional teaching methods can't get the job done; they only frustrate the student.

Creating the Concept

For nonverbal thinkers, an important element has been left out of the education process: creativity. The creative process and the learning process, if not identical, are so closely related that they are inseparable. If there is one thing dyslexics love to do, it is to exercise their creativity.

It's only my opinion, but I think learning should be fun.

People seem to learn more easily, thoroughly and quickly when the subject is interesting and entertaining. As human beings, we enjoy pleasurable experiences and seem to have a natural capacity to remember them.

If we want the dyslexic to think with the meaning of a trigger word, the dyslexic should be allowed to *create* a personal mental picture that accurately shows the meaning. Showing a dyslexic a photograph that represents the meaning of a trigger word may be better than saying the definition, but unless the dyslexic actually creates the picture, not much will be gained.

The Davis Symbol Mastery Procedure consists of having the person create the meaning of a word or symbol as a three-dimensional picture. The person makes a clay model that illustrates the meaning of the word or symbol, accompanied by a clay figure of the word itself. For abstract words such as articles and prepositions, the clay models take the form of scenarios illustrating the concept or relationship represented. The person then says the word aloud and makes up sentences using it. By creating

How I Finally Learned the Alphabet

As a child, I had a problem called autism. It is like super-dyslexia, only with more severe disorientations triggered by auditory stimuli. At the age of twelve, I still hadn't learned the alphabet. Even the "Alphabet Song" couldn't get me past the letter "G."

The alphabet was displayed on a banner across the top of a blackboard at school, but I couldn't keep the letters straight. They always seemed to be turning upside down, reversing into mirror images or appearing in a different place.

One thing I could do was make highly detailed models of things from muddy clay I dug out of a small pit in the backyard. One day, I formed a *D*, an *F* and an *O* from ropes of clay and left them to dry on the ground. The next day, the *D*, *F* and *O* on the banner at school held still and stayed in their correct places. When I went home to check, I discovered that I had made only one mistake: My clay *F* was backward. That was easy to fix by flipping it over.

I had memorized the shapes of a few more letters that day, so I proceeded to make them out of clay. I kept adding a couple of letters each day until I had all 26, arranged in the order they appeared on the chart. Once I had done this, I knew the forms of all the capital letters and their correct sequence.

This experience helped me develop the Davis Symbol Mastery Procedure.

the conceptual picture on a tabletop, with a clay model, and making the sound of the word, the person gains the ability to think with that word or symbol in both verbal and nonverbal modes. The Davis Symbol Mastery procedures are described fully in chapters 33 and 35.

Once all the trigger words that stimulate disorientation are mastered with Symbol Mastery, the dyslexic will no longer have a learning disability. The root causes of the disability have been eliminated, so compulsive solutions are no longer being triggered. "Old solution" behaviors will continue for a while, but over time the dyslexic will experience easier ways of doing things. The old solution will be dropped, and the one that works better will be adopted. The new solution will not be compulsive like the old solution because it is done consciously, with full understanding. At this point, it would be safe to say that the person's dyslexia is corrected.

PART TWO

Little P.D.

A Developmental Theory of Dyslexia

Every time we teach a child something,
we prevent him from inventing it himself.

—Jean Piaget

CHAPTER 13

How Dyslexia Happens

Apparently, some people are born with a genetic code that enables them to utilize the part of their brain that alters and creates perceptions. Being born with this genetic code doesn't give them dyslexia, it only makes it possible for them to develop it. This theory explains why dyslexia seems to follow family lines and why many experts consider it to be hereditary.

Developing dyslexia involves some rather complex steps, and the timing has to be precise. In fact, developing dyslexia is so complicated that it's a wonder anyone can do it.

An Early Start

A dyslexic didn't start to develop dyslexia in third grade or first grade, or even in kindergarten. The process began long before that. The dyslexic started using the special talent that brings about dyslexia possibly as early as three months of age.

Probably it is between the ages of three and six months that dyslexics begin the development of their special abilities, skills and deficiencies. I speculate that if an infant starts using the distortion function of the brain before the age of three months, the resulting problems will be far more severe than dyslexia. This might result in such inaccurate perceptions that the person could not relate to the outside word normally. The person would probably be labeled *autistic* or *developmentally disabled.*

The Potential Dyslexic in Infancy

Psychologists say a three-month-old infant is just beginning to recognize facial features. That means the infant can focus the eyes and control convergence of the two mental images they produce; otherwise it couldn't even see a face. Although a three-month-old can see, the child hasn't yet learned to control its neck muscles in order to look in a certain direction. The child simply sees whatever happens to move into its field of vision.

Let's create a scenario of a Potential Dyslexic, P.D. for short. Let's make little P.D. three months old and put him in a crib. From his perspective, all little P.D. can see is the end of a chest of drawers with someone's elbow sticking out past the edge.

If little P.D. happens to trigger the brain cells that alter his perception, he will no longer see what his eyes see; he will see something else. At that point, if P.D. is curious as to who the elbow belongs to, it would be very easy for him to simply add the other features to the elbow and see the face of the person. When he sees the face, he can recognize whether or not it's the person that feeds him.

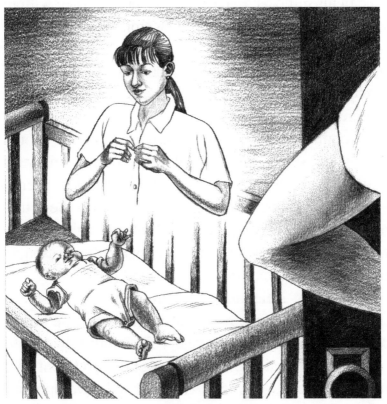

When little P.D. disorients his perceptions, a glimpse of his mother's elbow provides him with a complete mental image of her. Once he exercises this ability successfully, he continues using it to explore his environment.

We don't fully understand what little P.D. just did. It seems to border on the supernatural, but that is only because we don't fully understand the nature of intuitive thought. Perhaps it was a subliminal mental association between the arm P.D. had just seen and his mental image of the face he had already seen.

Through whatever means, little P.D. actually saw a face in his mind as real as the one he would see with his eyes, and recognized it as the face of his mother.

This mental talent P.D. uses to recognize an object never seems to make a mistake. His "self-created" perceptions always seem to be accurate as to what or whom the object is.

Of course, there's another way to recognize another person by seeing only an elbow: through analytical reasoning and logic. P.D. doesn't have those conscious skills yet. Children don't begin to develop them until about the age of three years. P.D. didn't think about anything or go through the process of elimination, he just *used* disorientation.

So here is little three-month-old P.D. recognizing things in his environment that he shouldn't be able to recognize for three more years. This ability he has for recognizing real objects in his environment will influence the rest of his early childhood development.

Little P.D.'s other early childhood skills may develop more rapidly than normal, or they may be delayed. He will probably have some areas of accelerated development and some of delayed development, both stemming from the same cause: his ability to mentally complete fragmentary perceptions.

The Visual Buffer

Dr. Stephen Kosslyn, a Harvard University psychologist, says that the visual center of the brain contains a "visual buffer" where images are perceived and sent to the upper conceptual centers of the brain for processing. The converse also occurs when thoughts and stored visual images are sent back to the visual buffer. There they are perceived as visual images for purposes of recognition by what he also calls "the mind's eye."

The real and mental images can be combined and confused, he says. An example is the fact that eyewitnesses of crimes or accidents often believe they saw what their expectations told them to see—not what actually happened.

Kosslyn, S. M. (1994). *Image and Brain: The Resolution of the Imagery Debate.* Cambridge, Mass.: MIT Press.

CHAPTER 14

The Two-Year-Old and the Kitten

Let's look at the next stage of little P.D.'s development, beginning at around the age of two years. He is becoming very curious. Too curious, his parents say. He is getting into everything. Little P.D. has explored every inch of his environment, including under the sinks, inside the cabinets, inside the laundry hamper and every place else that it was possible for him to get into. He has dumped everything out of every box and bottle he could get his hands on and probably tasted most of it. He is so environmentally aware that his parents can't bring something new into the house without his finding it almost immediately.

Let's see how well little P.D.'s dyslexic talents are progressing by giving him a little white kitten. But instead of handing it to him, let's curl it up into a tight white ball and put it in the corner of the living room.

Then let's have little P.D. toddle into the room. He doesn't get more than three steps into the room before his attention is drawn to the ball of fur in the corner. As soon as his eyes track to it, he begins to totter, rocking back and forth. In less than a second he exclaims, "Kitty!" and heads for the ball of fluff in the corner.

How could a two-year-old child recognize a white ball of fur as a kitten, not as a bunny or some furry toy? The same way he could recognize his mother almost two years earlier. As soon as his eyes tracked to the object and he didn't recognize what it was, he experienced a feeling of confusion. The feeling of confusion triggered the part of the brain that alters his perception. He momentarily lost his sense of balance. The room became silent. His inner clock skipped a beat. During that instant, his perceptual talent allowed him to look at the ball of fur from every angle and direction.

But the kitten was rolled up tightly. A ball of fur is only a ball of fur from every view. So how could he recognize it as a kitten?

If little P.D. has ever seen something come apart, like groceries out of a grocery bag or a gift being unwrapped, that process has already been incorporated into his thinking process. So after he used his perceptual ability to look at the ball of fur from every possible direction, it began to come apart in his mental image. Out came a paw, then another paw and a tail, then out popped the head and P.D. recognized the kitten.

As soon as the recognition occurred, P.D.'s feeling of confusion disappeared. The disorientation function of his brain shut off. At that moment P.D. regained his sense of balance, so he didn't fall down, he only tottered. At the same moment his hearing turned on again, his internal clock started ticking again, and he dived for the kitten in the corner.

P.D. isn't aware that his brain just looked at possibly 2,000 views of what that ball of fur might be. It happened too fast. The most little P.D. could be aware of would be a blurring of his vision for two blinks of his eyes, a sensation of floating, or a feeling of sinking. He may even have felt a little queasy. But the entire episode was over so fast that he hardly noticed.

By the age of two, little P.D. is automatically and unconsciously using the function of disorientation to recognize objects in his environment. He is rewarded for using it, because the process never seems to make a mistake.

CHAPTER 15

Ages Three to Five

What happens between the ages of three and five will make it possible for little P.D. to be more intelligent than normal, but will also create the potential for him to develop a learning disability.

In typical childhood development, the skills for analytical reasoning and logic should begin to develop at around the age of three. These are the skills for *consciously* recognizing people by seeing elbows, and kittens by seeing white balls of fur. Children who need these skills begin to develop them. But little P.D. already has a system that is faster and more accurate than analytical reasoning and logic ever could be. He has no need for those skills at all, so they don't develop.

Children who need the skills of analytical reasoning and logic must also start to develop their skills of verbal conceptualization, because reasoning and logic are language-based processes. These forms of thinking occur in the same patterns as sentences. So a typical child must use the speech and language center on the left side of the brain in his or her thought process.

This explains why verbal conceptualization is many times slower than nonverbal conceptualization: The speech and language center of the brain must, of necessity, operate at the maximum intelligible speed of speech—at most, perhaps 250 words per minute, or about 4 words per second. The result is that the typical child's thinking process is dramatically slowing down, while P.D.'s mind continues to race along at full speed.

P.D. has, of course, learned to understand spoken language and can talk. In fact, he sometimes tries to talk as fast as he can think, and his mouth can't keep up with his mind. When he is trying to say something he considers important, his speech speeds up so much that the words run together. What his parents hear is an unintelligible garble of sounds. They worry that he may be developing a stutter.

"Slow down, honey," says his mother. "You're talking so fast I can't understand what you're saying." To P.D., who is trying to describe a thought he is visualizing, her speech sounds agonizingly slow.

It's as if she is speaking at the rate of less than one . . . word . . . per . . . second.

Estimates of the speed differential between verbal and nonverbal conceptualization range from 400 to

2,000 times faster when people use the nonverbal mode. The reality is probably somewhere in between.

The process of developing verbal conceptualization skills (thinking with the sound of language) can take up to two years. Once it fully develops, it will become the primary thinking mode of most children. So by the age of five, at about the time kindergarten begins, typical children have already begun to think with the sounds of words. This may be slow, but it will come in handy when they begin learning how to read.

Meanwhile, although he has heard people say things and has said quite a lot himself, P.D. hasn't ever *heard* one of his own thoughts. He has been too busy thinking with pictures—a thought process that happens so fast, he doesn't even notice he's doing it.

CHAPTER 16

The First Day of School

To see the effect of nonverbal thinking on little P.D., let's make him six years old and send him to first grade. No matter how prepared he was for this day, and no matter how enthusiastically he was looking forward to it, the reality is terrifying.

He is in a strange place. There he sits. He's scared to death. He would rather be anywhere else in the world than where he is.

Now let's have a strange lady go up to the blackboard with a piece of chalk and write the letters *C-A-T.* She turns around and says, "Who knows what this is?" Some of the other kids have already learned the word, but P.D. doesn't know. Even when they say "cat," he makes no connection. The lines don't form anything like his mental picture of a cat.

When he looked at the lines on the board and didn't

recognize what they were, he experienced the feeling of confusion. By this time, confusion *automatically* triggers the area of his brain that alters his perception. Within a blink of his eyes, his brain looks at the word in at least 40 different configurations. He perceives the word forward, backward, upside down both ways and floating in space from various perspectives.

Then, in another blink, because it still has not been recognized, the word will be pulled apart and reassembled in every possible configuration just like the image of the white, furry cat when he was two. Only this time it won't work.

P.D. isn't aware that his brain just took in all those conflicting pieces of data. The most he could have noticed was that things may have gotten blurry for two blinks of his eyes. He may have had the sensation of floating or sinking, and he may have felt a little sick to his stomach. But most of all, he felt confused.

Stumped

For the first time in his life, P.D.'s special method for recognizing things didn't work. It not only failed to recognize the word and get rid of the confusion, it made the word at least 40 times more confusing. He was trying to understand the word not as a symbol, but as an object.

Had the teacher shown him a real cat, P.D. would

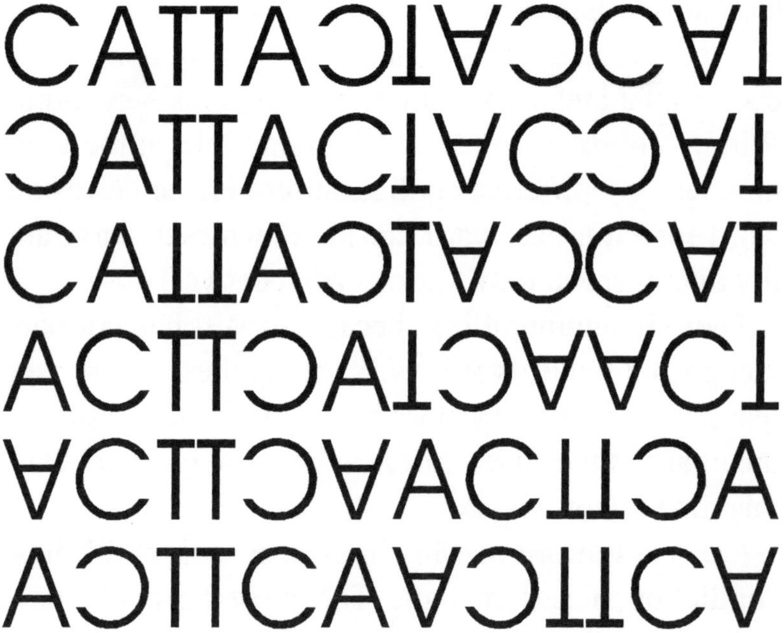

CATTACIAƆCAT
ƆATTACIAƆƆAT
CA�ART ꓘꓘ
ACTTƆAꓘ
ꓘCTTƆꓘ
ꓘƆTTCAꓘ
ATCƆTAꓘ
CTAATƆ
AꓘCƆꓘ
ꓘTƆCT

Forty dyslexic variations of the word CAT.

have recognized it within two blinks of his eyes, even if it were rolled up into a tight ball of fur. He could have done that three years before he entered the classroom. But the teacher didn't show him a cat; she showed him the word *CAT.* The same function his brain would perform to recognize the object almost instantly produced multiple dyslexic distortions of the word but with no resolution of his confusion.

If we look at this from a different perspective, P.D. just put at least 40 pieces of data into his mental computer. Thirty-nine pieces of data were incorrect.

The only method little P.D. has for determining the correct data is the process of elimination. So without anyone showing him or telling him how to do it, he eventually happens upon it by himself.

Sometime after he begins doing the process of elimination, the teacher will come by and say something like, "P.D., honey, you're not supposed to guess. Here, try . . ." What he was doing looked exactly like guessing, but it wasn't.

By the time little P.D. does all the things he must do to recognize the word *CAT*, he will have performed at least 4,000 times more computations in his brain than the other children. It's true that he can think between 400 and 2,000 times faster than most other children. But because he has to do at least 4,000 times more, he will appear very *slow.*

Invalidation

The teacher's remark may seem trivial, but it is essential to the creation of dyslexia. Until someone tells P.D. that his method of dealing with incorrect data and confusion is wrong, he won't manifest the emotional reactions associated with the learning disability of dyslexia.

If the invalidation happens in kindergarten, he will develop dyslexia in kindergarten. If it doesn't happen until third grade, he won't have dyslexia until third grade. The struggle to comprehend will be there, but

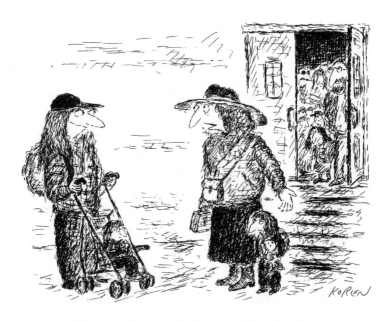

"Can you believe this is happening to me?
Her scores are very low in self-esteem."

P.D. won't become aware that he is different from other children, and won't lose his sense of self-esteem.

Even little P.D. isn't aware that he is using the process of elimination. He isn't aware that he has at least 39 pieces of incorrect data for every three-letter word he has failed to recognize.

He isn't aware that the process he is using to eliminate incorrect data is the only one available to him if he wants to arrive at a correct answer. At his age, he doesn't know the difference between guessing and making mistakes. As far as he is concerned, he is making mistakes.

No one likes making mistakes, so P.D. has the natural human reaction to mistakes. He gets upset. Before long, his emotional reactions upset the teacher. The teacher in turn upsets the school administration, and they upset P.D.'s parents.

Someone will eventually tell the parents that P.D. is immature or a slow developer, or some such thing. They usually don't use the words *dumb* or *stupid*, but the message comes across clearly.

Once P.D. gets upset about making his mistakes, everyone is bound to get upset with him, so he becomes increasingly frustrated. He is frustrated because these word things should be easy, as easy as everything else. But they aren't; they're impossible.

At this point, P.D. has acquired the emotional distress he needs to become a full-fledged dyslexic.

CHAPTER 17

The Age of Disability

At about the age of nine, when he is in third grade, young P.D. reaches his limit of frustration. If he doesn't figure out a way to get over, under, around or through his problem with words, he'll be stuck in third grade for the rest of his life. By now school has become torture, so he is desperate.

P.D. begins to solve his problem. He finds mental tricks and gimmicks like rote memorization and associations of sounds, songs, rhymes—and worst of all, concentration. These allow him to function in the world of words. Everyone is happy for him now that he is finally making some progress. He has finally started to learn his lessons, but the lessons have little to do with genuine learning. The lessons he learns will comprise a lifelong disability. They are compulsive behaviors. At best, they may enable him to get by in school as a "slow" student who "tries hard."

P.D. has begun the process of accumulating his "old solutions." He is beginning to change a limitation into a disability. It was a limitation because he had to perform thousands of times more computations than the other students just to recognize three-letter words. It will become a disability because he has no control over his "old solutions." They control him.

If P.D. finds himself in a special education class, he will have the opportunity to acquire more of these ruses than if he stayed in a regular class. Special ed teachers are usually very good at passing their own "old solutions" along to their students. This can make it appear that children are making a little progress. Unfortunately, special ed class also lowers P.D.'s self-esteem even more. Being there convinces him beyond a doubt that he is lacking in intelligence. In first grade, they only hinted about his stupidity. Now it has been confirmed.

If he isn't put into a special education class, P.D. might be held back a year or even two years during elementary school. Being a year or two older than the other kids might be embarrassing in the classroom, but his size and advanced development in non-academic areas may provide him with advantages in physical education, music and art, as well as recess and after-school activities.

To compensate and find some form of self-esteem, P.D. may adopt any number of interests, none of which has to do with reading and writing. It could be a sport, visual arts, music or acting. It could be rebellion. If he decides to be a "bad kid" as a defense, and gives his parents and teachers trouble, he may discover he has a real talent for delinquency.

During his teenage years, his talent for sizing up a situation and motivating others may provide opportunities for leadership, whether in a school club, sports, a part-time job or a gang.

It would be easy to blame the problem of dyslexia on the educational system, but according to the basic premise of dyslexia presented here, it's clear that the dyslexic created the condition. P.D. is responsible for all the actions that produced the learning disability. He alone learned to distort his perceptions. If we try to put that responsibility anywhere else, his problems will never be completely resolved. Of course he was unaware of his actions, but that doesn't alter the fact that only P.D. can learn to undo what he has done.

The Dyslexic Grows Up

To P.D., school classes that involve reading and writing are mental torture chambers. He learns much of what is taught in art, music and science, because the teachers in those classes rely on verbal instruction and demonstration. But his written test scores are low, even in the courses he enjoys. Since everyone says education is important, P.D. completes as much school as he can tolerate. He may drop out of high school and get a job that allows him to use his excellent mechanical abilities. He may stay in high school and excel at sports, art or acting. If he's lucky, he may find a girlfriend to help him with English papers.

Later, he may struggle through college and go into business, even though his grade school reading level forces him to operate on a semi-illiterate basis wherever written communications are concerned.

Still Using the Talents

Whatever else P.D. does, he does not lose the initial gift he developed of looking at an object or situation and "just knowing" what it is. As he continues to observe the world, he also develops a keen, intuitive understanding of how things work. He is imaginative and inventive. He is visually and kinesthetically oriented. He is able to think on his feet and react quickly. He is a good athlete, conversationalist, salesperson or storyteller. If his self-esteem drops to a low enough level, he may become socially inept. Even so, he will find some way to maintain at least a little self-esteem, even if it is at the emotional expense of others.

Still, he does have a low opinion of himself, because he has spent at least half of his life hearing people describe him explicitly or implicitly as stupid or handicapped. He secretly hides his inability to read well, and invents ever more tricks and gimmicks to beat the system of the written word.

A Discovery

In 1980, I was lucky enough to discover how to correct the severe perceptual distortions that had been my everyday reality for 38 years.

I was working as a sculptor when another artist wrote and asked me about my sculpting technique. His letter was so filled with praise that I began the laborious process of composing a response. Hours later, after carefully getting my thoughts down, I discovered that the letter was totally illegible—just a bunch of meaningless scrawls that nobody could ever read.

Months later, it occurred to me that when I wrote the letter, I had been focusing on my creative process. I wondered if this was what had made my dyslexia worse. The engineer in me reasoned that if my dyslexia could be changed by something I was doing mentally, it could not possibly be a structural problem but must be a functional problem. Thus, there had to be something I could do mentally to correct my dyslexia. This was my first step as a researcher in the field of learning disabilities.

Three days later, I managed to figure out how to correct my perceptual distortions. I went to the library, picked up *Treasure Island*, and, for the first time in my life, read a book cover to cover in just a few hours.

Since then, I have worked at developing techniques based on what I discovered. I have had the pleasure of training hundreds of Davis Facilitators around the world, who have helped tens of thousands of children and adults learn to make the words—and the world—stand still.

Along the way, P.D. may take seminars and self-improvement courses that attempt to "cure" or help him cope with his disability. Some might help. Some might introduce more compulsive solutions in the form of conditioned behaviors. Some might help him learn things that have nothing to do with reading or writing. Most likely, he will find ways to simply do what he can do well and avoid what he can't do. If he has a job that requires him to fill out reports, he will find a way to get someone else to do them.

Someday, he might discover that he is talented at a visual art like sculpting. In fact, because he can visualize the form he wants to sculpt, he can do it effortlessly. To make a bust, all he has to do is place an image of someone's head inside a block of wood or clay and carve the excess material from around the edges. Or he can put an image of the head on a table and fill it with material as if it were an invisible mold.

This last specific example is from my own life. In fact, many of little P.D.'s experiences were really those of little R.D.—Ron Davis.

PART THREE

The Gift

The Gifted Vintner

Mark was eight when he came to the Reading Research Council. He had struggled through second grade, but was performing below first grade level. His teachers had suggested that he be tested for neurological damage. This didn't make sense to his mother. Even though he was doing poorly in school, she knew he had special gifts in many areas.

Mark's family were fourth-generation vintners. Since he was four, his grandfather took him along to the vineyards and the winery. To Mark, the art and science of wine making were play. By age six, he could tell when the time was right to pick and press the grapes. He just knew when the sugar content was right, or when the acid in the skins wasn't. He could tell when fermentation was complete, when to move the wines from vats to barrels, and from barrels to bottles. If you asked him how he knew, he would just tap the side of his head with his finger. His great-grandfather had had the same sense for the grapes, considered the greatest gift a vintner can possess.

When Mark's mother read a story in the local newspaper about our work, the list of dyslexia symptoms I had given to the reporter caught her eye. One was intuitive thinking ability, where some dyslexics just know things without conscious understanding of how or why.

She explained, "The symptoms in the article fit with so many things I'd noticed about Mark when he was little. He rarely cried. He walked before he crawled. He started talking much earlier than all my friends' babies. He could remember events perfectly, even those that happened when he was an infant. Yet he could hardly say the alphabet or spell his own name. I had never heard dyslexia described that way before, but it fit my son like a glove. Until then I had no idea that Mark's special abilities and his learning problems were related."

CHAPTER 18

Understanding the Talent

Like the negative side of dyslexia, where no two people have the same disabilities, the gift of dyslexia is different for each person. There are, however, general characteristics that all dyslexics have in common.

Like its negative aspect, the gift of dyslexia is developmental. It has to grow. It must be created by the dyslexic. Over time it changes. Often it doesn't fully develop until the dyslexic has been out of school for a number of years. Perhaps the intervening years are a sort of recovery period.

The eventual gift of dyslexia will be the gift of *mastery*. The dyslexic will be able to master many skills faster than the average person could comprehend or understand them.

The gift of mastery is an accumulation of various characteristics of the individual's basic abilities. It begins with the characteristic of nonverbal thought.

Picture Thinking

The primary thought process of the dyslexic is a nonverbal picture thinking mode that occurs at 32 pictures per second. In a second, a verbal thinker could have between two and five thoughts (individual words conceptualized) while a picture thinker would have 32 (individual pictures conceptualized). Mathematically, this works out to between six and ten times as many thoughts.

There is also the principle expressed by the old adage "A picture is worth a thousand words." A picture thinker could think a single picture of a concept that might require hundreds or thousands of words to describe. Einstein's theory of relativity came to him in a *daydream* in which he traveled beside a beam of light. His vision lasted only seconds, yet spawned scores of textbooks that attempt to explain it. To Einstein, the concept was simple; to the average person, it is nearly incomprehensible.

Picture thinking is estimated to be, overall, 400 to 2,000 times faster than verbal thinking. Obviously, it varies with the complexity of the individual pictures. But there is more to it than just a difference in speed. Picture thinking is more thorough, deeper and more comprehensive.

Verbal thought is linear in time, performed by making sentences one word at a time, whereas picture thinking is evolutionary. The picture grows as the mental process adds more subconcepts to the overall concept.

Pictured thoughts are as thorough or deep as these mental pictures are accurate in portraying the meanings of the words that the person would use to describe the same thoughts.

We could say pictured thoughts are of *substance* while verbal thoughts are *significant sound.*

Intuition

The only drawback to picture thinking is that the person doing it is not aware of the individual pictures as they occur. It happens too fast. The *incidence of awareness* is the amount of time it takes for something to register consciously in the awareness of the individual. In humans it is fairly consistent at 1/25 of a second. In other words, a stimulus must be present for 1/25 of a second in order to register in the person's consciousness.

If a stimulus is present longer than 1/25 of a second, we are aware of it. This is called *cognizance.* If a stimulus is present for less than 1/25 of a second, but longer than 1/36 of a second, it falls into the category called *subliminal.* Our brain gets it, but we aren't aware of what it got. If it is part of a continuum, it fuses with the pictures that precede and follow. If a stimulus isn't present for at least 1/36 of a second, we don't even get it subliminally. It went by too fast for our brain to catch it at all.

Picture thinking seems to be consistently happening at about 32 pictures per second, or a frequency of 1/32 of a second, the same speed as the flicker-fusion rate of the eye. In other words, the eye's shutter speed.

This is somewhat faster than the incidence of awareness at 1/25 of a second, but slower than the subliminal limit of 1/36 of a second. So picture thinking falls within the subliminal band.

The person's brain gets the thought, but the person isn't consciously aware of it. As a result, we can begin to understand *intuition*, because picture thinking is the same as intuitive thinking. The person becomes aware of the product of the thought process as soon as it occurs, but is not aware of the process as it is happening. The person knows the answer without knowing why it is the answer.

Many dyslexics find a way to bring the subliminal thought process into their awareness. If they think of something interesting, they can disorient into the thought and watch the individual pictures as they occur. When they do this, it is called a *daydream*. Parents and teachers are very critical of daydreaming, but they shouldn't be. In fact, they should encourage it at every opportunity. Daydreaming is the process of genius, as Einstein and others have proven time and again.

Multidimensional Thought

Disorientation adds dimension to the thought process. The thinking is no longer subliminal, or only in pictures. Multidimensional thought uses all the senses.

The Incidence of Awareness

TV frames appear on the screen at a speed of 30 frames per second, fast enough to trick our eyes into seeing smooth motion. Modern movies, projected at 24 frames per second, trick our eyes most of the time, but occasionally make the wheels of a stagecoach appear to spin backward. Old silent movies, filmed at sixteen frames per second, appear noticeably jerky. Our brains can easily catch the jumps between individual pictures.

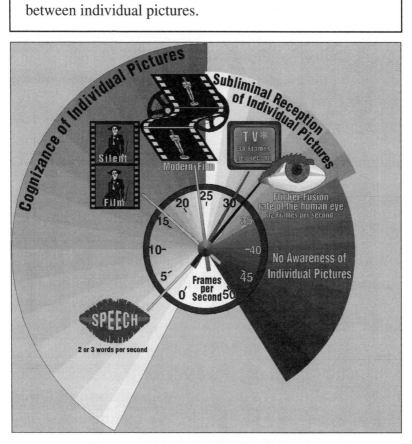

In most countries outside North America, television runs at 25 frames per second.

When a disorientation has occurred, the brain no longer sees what the eyes are looking at, but what the person is thinking, *as though* the eyes were seeing it. The brain no longer hears what the ears are hearing, but what the person is thinking, *as though* the ears were hearing it. The body no longer feels what its senses are feeling, but what the person is thinking, and so on.

One aspect of multidimensional thinking is the ability of the thinker to experience thoughts as realities.

Reality is what the person perceives it to be, and the disorientation alters the perception. The person's thoughts become the person's perceptions, so the thoughts are *reality* to that individual.

A Creative Process

If "necessity is the mother of invention," then multidimensional thinking must be its father. This concept helps us understand how Leonardo da Vinci could conceptualize a submarine 300 years before the invention of a device that could pump the water out of it. We see how he could envision a helicopter 400 years before there was an engine that could power one. There is little doubt Leonardo experienced flight and underwater travel hundreds of years before they became realities. His multidimensional ability allowed him to experience his thoughts as realities and draw the results for everyone else to see.

Of course, there were probably people in Leonardo's day who considered these ideas crazy.

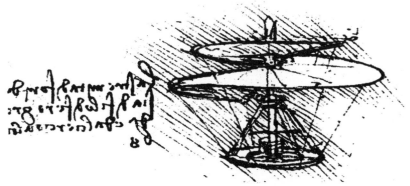

Leonardo visualized human-powered flight in this helicopter sketch. It is described by a note in the "mirror image" handwriting he used in his notebooks.

On the darker side, we can also begin to understand why mental institutions have numerous residents who are absolutely convinced they are Jesus Christ or Napoleon. Their problem is that they cannot distinguish between imaginary reality and the reality shared by most people.

CHAPTER 19

Curiosity

From as early as three months of age, a dyslexic has used disorientation to recognize objects in the environment. This ability is extremely accurate, seeming never to err. By the time a dyslexic is two years old, the disorientations have become automatic, occurring whenever the person encounters confusion.

The ability to recognize objects at such an early age makes dyslexics highly aware of the environment. As a result, dyslexic infants begin "getting into things" as soon as they are able to. The drive to become mobile is very strong. It is common for dyslexic children to begin walking months before child development books say they are supposed to.

It is common for parents to be driven to their wits' end trying to figure out ways to keep their dyslexic children *in* the places they want them, and *out* of places where they don't want them.

The Crawling Treatment

One of the stranger treatments for dyslexia, from the 1950s, sprang from the observation that children who later developed dyslexia had often begun to walk before they could crawl. The treatment was to make the dyslexics crawl around on the floor until the dyslexia went away. Of course it didn't work, but crawling therapy was added to many treatment programs for dyslexia, and is still practiced in some today.

The reaction of a mother who has just discovered her two-year-old child under the kitchen sink emptying the contents of all the boxes and bottles is understandable. This is dangerous behavior. Who knows what the child might have eaten? Even after a cooler head has prevailed, it is a behavior that must be changed.

We can't expect a child of this age to respond to rational arguments. Disciplining the child isn't the answer either, because the child is responding to an urge stronger than normal and one that usual disciplinary procedures will not correct. Besides, if we really understood what the child was doing, we wouldn't want to change it. So childproofing the kitchen and bathroom cabinets and putting plastic covers over doorknobs would be a better solution than spankings.

The dyslexic child isn't getting into things just to upset the parents. The child is responding to an urge that will eventually become part of the gift of dyslexia.

The seed that has begun to grow is *curiosity.* Curiosity is a stronger force than gravity. If it weren't, there wouldn't be airplanes. Curiosity is more important than knowledge; it is the root of knowledge. Without it there wouldn't be any such thing as knowledge.

Most importantly, curiosity is the dynamic force behind creativity. Without creativity, mankind would still be living in caves.

CHAPTER 20

Creativity

Creativity is what sets mankind above other life-forms. Some believe that God, the creator, made man in his image. If this is so, man in the image of God must be creative.

In the dyslexic, the creative urge is profoundly stronger than in individuals who do not possess the dyslexic's basic abilities. Because of *picture thinking*, *intuitive thought*, *multidimensional thought* and *curiosity*, the dyslexic's creativity is greatly enhanced.

Creativity allows us to conceive of things that don't actually exist. From that experience, we can bring new things into existence. All original ideas stem from the creative process.

We think of creativity as invention or innovation. That is correct, but on a more basic level, creativity is the means by which real learning takes place.

Conditioning is a very rudimentary form of learning. When we train a dog or a seal to do tricks, we condition the animal through rewards or penalties to behave in a desired manner. Humans can also be conditioned in this way, but it is much more difficult. Often the conditioning isn't effective.

Because of creativity, humans learn on a much higher level. The act of reasoning is a function of creativity. Logic is a product of creativity. Reasoning and logic are the foundations of learning. If we touch something that burns our fingers, it is with reasoning and logic we figure out why we shouldn't touch it again. We *learned* not to touch it.

In chapter 15, I mentioned that dyslexic children often haven't developed their skills in reasoning and logic by the time they start school. What they have developed is a variation of these skills that does not follow the linear model of verbal thought. Their analytical reasoning and logic is comparative, using pictures instead of words. This method might be great for figuring out the helical structure of DNA, but could be useless in attempting to do a math story problem in fifth grade.

Sometimes, like autistic savants, dyslexics can "see" the answers to math problems without using pen and paper. This is actually a highly developed form of reasoning. They solved the problem whether or not they bothered to go through the conventional steps. Often, investigation reveals that they have developed highly creative mathematical shortcuts.

If the creative process and the human learning process are not the exact same process, they are so closely related that they cannot be separated.

Assuming a dyslexic is inherently more creative than the average person, the dyslexic should also be able to *learn* more in less time. Theoretically this is true, but things may appear otherwise to educators and parents.

The probable reason is that so much education is done on the *conditioning* level. The child is told to go through a series of rote steps without seeing any personal benefit in arriving at a solution.

Dyslexia shouldn't be called a learning disability. It should more accurately be called a *conditioning liability*.

In real-life situations, such as on-the-job training, the arts and athletics, dyslexics do learn more in less time than the average person. In fact, when learning is presented experientially, dyslexics can master many things faster than the average person can comprehend them.

Spots in the Air

Until the age of thirteen, I was disoriented so much of the time that I was considered retarded. Today, I would be classified as autistic. Consequently, I have very few "real" memories of my childhood. But I don't doubt that the following incident, related to me by my mother, is true.

When I was in the fourth grade, my math teacher was puzzled by the fact that, while I couldn't work out simple problems, I could instantly come up with the answer to complex algebraic equations. One day he discussed this with my mother and asked me, "If X is one and Y is seven, what is two Y minus X?"

I instantly answered, "Thirteen." When asked how I got the answer, I said I saw it. When asked what it looked like, I touched two spots in the air, then touched three more spots under those.

The math teacher mentioned that he had heard of people called "savants" who could do this sort of thing.

"You mean idiot savants?" asked my mother indignantly. She chewed out the teacher for calling me an idiot, grabbed me by the arm and marched me out of school. After that, I was taken out of the class and not allowed to take any more math until the ninth grade, when I took algebra.

In algebra, I correctly answered every problem in the book, every problem the teacher put on the blackboard and every problem on the tests. Yet I failed the class. The teacher explained that the purpose of the class wasn't just to get right answers; it was to learn how to do the problems. I hadn't done a single one of them. All I had done was write down the answers.

CHAPTER 21

The Gift of Mastery

The gift of dyslexia is the gift of mastery.

When people have mastered something, they have learned it so well they can do it without thinking about what they are doing. Mastering something is *really* learning it. If the creative process and the learning process are the same, then when someone has mastered something, that person has *created* the knowledge it takes to do it.

All real knowledge is experiential. It is a mistake to confuse the memorization of data with the understanding of data. And it is a bigger mistake to confuse the understanding of data with knowledge.

When someone has an experience, that person has the knowledge of that experience. If the person then wishes to write that knowledge in a book, the knowledge must be converted into data. When someone else reads the book, the reader doesn't gain the knowledge, but only the data. If the reader understands the data, he or she will only understand the experience conceptually. But if the reader *really* wants the knowledge, it will be necessary to have an actual experience similar to that of the author.

If a person wanted to learn how to ride a bicycle, that person could get some books on riding bicycles. After studying all the data in the books, the person might *understand* the principles of riding a bicycle. If the person mistakenly thinks he or she knows how to ride a bicycle, and tries, the experience will quickly demonstrate the difference between *understanding* and *knowing* how to ride the bicycle.

The experience of being on the bicycle gives the rider the opportunity to *create* the act of riding a bicycle. As the person creates riding a bicycle, the person is learning how to ride a bicycle. At first there will be a lot of experimenting, thinking and remembering. As the actual experiences are created, less conscious effort will be needed. When the person can ride automatically, without any experimenting, thinking and remembering, the person has mastered riding the bicycle.

This is easy to comprehend for physical skills like riding a bicycle or driving a car, but not so apparent when it comes to learning a language, reading or math. However, the principle is the same.

When the same principle is applied to learning

language skills and math, dyslexics not only learn these skills, they master them. Davis Symbol Mastery is a process dyslexics can use to apply this principle to anything they want to learn.

Mastery is more than just fast learning. Mastery is a level of learning where conscious thought is no longer required. It is the ability to own the data learned as actual experience. When something is mastered, there is no need to worry about being able to remember it—it's probably impossible to forget.

When someone masters something, it becomes a part of that person. It becomes part of the individual's thought and creative process. It adds the quality of its essence to all subsequent thought and creativity of the individual.

PART FOUR

Doing Something About It

A Guide for Parents, Tutors and Educators

Orientation corrects perception.
Symbol Mastery corrects dyslexia.

—Ronald D. Davis

CHAPTER 22

How Can You Tell?

If you suspect that you or someone you care about has the gift of dyslexia, how can it be diagnosed? This seems like a simple, logical question that should have an equally simple, logical answer, but it isn't. If you consider for a moment what you have already read about dyslexia, the reasons for the difficulty will be apparent.

Diverse Symptoms, No Pathology

The traditional method for diagnosing a problem is to test the person and then study the results with either symptomatology or pathology.

Using symptomatology, the study of symptoms, to diagnose dyslexia can cause many problems. The first is that no two people with dyslexia ever exhibit the same symptoms. Until all of the people who have dyslexia add their symptoms to the list, we won't even know what all the symptoms might be. In addition, all the known symptoms of dyslexia can result from other causes, including physical disorders such as vision and inner-ear problems.

In pathology, the study of the nature of disease, the structural and functional changes in the body caused by disease are studied. The big drawback here is that dyslexia isn't a disease, but a self-created condition.

As the equipment for looking inside bodies becomes more and more sophisticated, there are anomalies we might expect to find, such as a slightly larger pineal gland and more large neurons, which would cause the corpus callosum to be slightly thicker. But considering dyslexia as a developmental process, these anomalies would be a result of the difference in the way the dyslexic's brain develops through use. Saying they cause dyslexia would be incorrect.

These hypothetical differences would also be present in anyone who has the gift of dyslexia, not just those who develop learning disabilities.

As a result, there is no definitive diagnostic test for dyslexia. This is probably the reason some psychologists and educators say, "There is no such thing as dyslexia." But there is.

If we look at the structure or anatomy of the learning disability known as dyslexia, we find that this sequence of development occurs:

1. **The individual encounters an unrecognized stimulus.** This could be a word (written or spoken), a symbol or an object that is not recognized.

2. **The lack of recognition causes a confusion, which stimulates disorientation.** The individual uses disorientation to mentally examine the stimulus from different points of view, in an attempt to bring about recognition. This usually works with real-life objects, but doesn't work at all with language, because it is composed of sonic or written symbols for ideas and concepts.

3. **The disorientation causes the assimilation of incorrect data.** The perspectives the individual examines mentally are registered in the brain as actual perceptions. Most of these perceptions are inaccurate.

4. **The assimilation of incorrect data causes the individual to make mistakes.** The individual cannot distinguish between correct and incorrect data, because both are registered in the brain as actual perceptions. The resulting mistakes are usually the first "symptoms" of dyslexia.

5. **The mistakes cause emotional reactions.** No one likes making mistakes. The individual is simply experiencing a human reaction. This, in turn, causes teachers and parents to react negatively.

6. **Emotional reactions bring about frustration.**
The frustration is a result of the cumulative
effects of mistakes and emotional reactions,
compounded by the negative responses of other
people.

7. **Solutions are created or adopted to solve
the problems stemming from the use of
disorientation in the recognition process.**
These solutions will be methods of seeming to
know things or of performing tasks. Each will
have worked at least once, and will be a
compulsive behavior. The person will use it
without even noticing. These "old solutions"
usually begin to accumulate at around age
nine.

8. **The learning disability is composed of
the compulsive solutions the individual
acquires.** Compulsive solutions are mental
crutches, rote memorizations, tricks or gimmicks the person uses to give the *appearance*
of understanding. They have little if anything
to do with actually learning or gaining
understanding of the material studied.

9. **These compulsive solutions are what disable
the learning process.** By using compulsive
solutions, a person might learn to "read" the
way a parrot learns to talk—without any
understanding of the content. Through a few

more roundabout mental processes, the person might be able to decipher some of the meaning of the material that is read. But using these solutions is a tedious process.

With this anatomy as a base, we can assess for the characteristics of the mental functions that eventually produce various levels of dyslexia: the ability to do nonverbal conceptualization and the ability to disorient the perceptions.

CHAPTER 23

Symptoms of Disorientation

Symptoms are the first things people notice that cause them to suspect a learning disability. We must be familiar with "known" symptoms, or at least understand the nature of the problem, before we can assess for it.

All of the symptoms of dyslexia are symptoms of disorientation. Dyslexia itself can't be definitively recognized, but disorientation can.

During a disorientation, a person's perceptions become distorted. What is mentally perceived as real is not in agreement with the true facts and conditions in the environment. The main senses that become distorted are vision, hearing, balance, movement and time. Common examples of disorientation include motion sickness, the sense of falling when on an escalator or at the edge of a cliff, "hearing things" and the false sense of motion people sometimes experience when they are sitting in a stopped vehicle and see another nearby vehicle move.

While a person is disoriented, he or she isn't perceiving the same "reality" as others, and is unaware that what is being perceived is not real.

Thousands of different learning disability symptoms can result from disorientation. The severity and degree to which each of the senses is affected varies from person to person, and from one time to another. The following are some of the most common symptoms of disorientation categorized by the sensory perceptions most affected:

Vision

- Shapes and sequences of letters or numbers appear changed or reversed.
- Spelling is incorrect or inconsistent.
- Words or lines are skipped when reading or writing.
- Letters and numbers appear to move, disappear, grow or shrink.
- Punctuation marks or capital letters are omitted, ignored or not seen.
- Words and letters are omitted, altered or substituted while reading or writing.

Hearing

- Some speech sounds are difficult to make.
- Digraphs such as *ch*, *th* and *sh* are mispronounced.
- "False" sounds are perceived.
- What is said does not appear to be listened to or heard.
- Sounds are perceived as quieter, louder, farther away or nearer than actual.

Balance/Movement

- Dizziness or nausea while reading
- Poor sense of direction
- Inability to sit still
- Difficulty with handwriting
- Problems with balance and coordination

Time

- Hyperactivity (being overactive)
- Hypoactivity (being underactive)
- Difficulty learning math concepts
- Difficulty being on time or telling time
- Excessive daydreaming
- Frequent loss of train of thought
- Trouble sequencing (putting things in the correct order)

Compulsive Solutions

There are hundreds of compensating behaviors, patterns and mental tricks a person can create or adopt as compulsive solutions to unresolved confusions that slow or stop the ability to learn. Here are some of the more common ones:

- Singing the "Alphabet Song" aloud or mentally
- Extreme concentration when reading
- Memorization
- Unusual body postures and motions
- Dependence on others
- Sounding out every letter of every word
- Avoidance

Any combination of the symptoms and behaviors in the five lists above may exist in one individual, while others may be entirely absent.

Ability Assessment

Besides finding symptoms that reveal the negative aspects of disorientation, we can also assess for the presence of four basic abilities shared by many dyslexics. These talents are usually part of the gift of dyslexia.

1. The ability to intentionally access the brain's perception-distortion function

2. The ability to consciously view mental images three-dimensionally and move around them in mental space

3. The ability to experience self-created mental images as real-world phenomena; in other words, being able to experience imagination as reality

4. A tendency or preference to think nonverbally by using pictures of concepts and ideas, with little or no internal monologue

If these are present, and the individual manifests symptoms of a learning disability, we can safely assume that the symptoms are a result of disorientation. We can use the results of our assessment to determine the best way to begin to resolve the disorientation.

Before we get into the step-by-step procedures of assessment and correction, one more concept needs definition. It explains what the person actually does in order to activate the disorientation function of the brain.

CHAPTER 24

The Mind's Eye

What I discovered in December 1980 came as a result of noticing that when I was at "my artistic best" I was also at "my dyslexic worst." Because my symptoms were not constant, this made me question the assumption that dyslexia stemmed from a structural deficit or dysfunction of the brain.

By examining how I viewed things while creating artistically, I discovered that during creative thinking, I was shifting the location of the viewpoint that looks at my mental images. I found that by playing with various locations for "what was doing the looking," I could intentionally increase and decrease the severity of my dyslexia symptoms.

Because I could find no term for "what was doing the looking," I at first coined the term "visio-awareness epicenter," or VAE. At the time, this seemed to be a technically correct assemblage of root word concepts, but I preferred something simpler. So I adopted the term "the mind's eye," which is defined in dictionaries as "the imagination."

Later, I discovered that what I termed "the mind's eye" was also the mental epicenter of other perceptions, such as sound and the senses of balance and motion. So a totally correct term might be "the mind's epicenter of perception." I have stuck with "the mind's eye" because it is an easier concept for people to grasp. This may be because vision is the predominant perception, and the one that usually gives dyslexics the most trouble.

A Mental Viewpoint

It is important to note that in the Davis procedures, one does not see, look at or sense anything *in*, *through* or *at* the mind's eye. One sees or looks *with*, *from* or *out of* the mind's eye.

Obviously, if you are looking *at* something, you have to be looking *from* somewhere. To put it another way, if you look out of your eyes, you don't see your own face. You can only see a mirror image of it or a photograph of it, but not the face itself, because that is where you are looking from. Similarly, the mind's eye cannot perceive itself. It can perceive only things outside itself, whether they exist in the mind as concepts or in the real world as objects.

When you look at a mental image such as an imagined event or a dream, the mind's eye is what you are looking with, from or out of.

Locating the Mind's Eye

The mind's eye does have a location. In fact, it has a multitude of possible locations. It is wherever its owner intends it, wishes it or perceives it to be. If this sounds like a supernatural or metaphysical concept, please remember that dyslexics are able to experience their mental images as actual perceptions. So if they place the mind's eye in a particular place, they gain the ability to experience their perceptions from that perspective.

When dyslexic people look at an alphabet letter and disorient, within a split second they see dozens of different views—from the top, the sides and the back of the letter. In other words, the mind's eye is mentally circling around the letter as though it were an object in three-dimensional space. It's like a helicopter buzzing around, doing surveillance on a building. This is the disorientation function hard at work, trying to recognize the object.

Is the mind's eye actually out there in the "real" world, circling around the letter and moving behind the page of the book? Is the person having an out-of-body experience? Or is the person's mind manufacturing the perceptual stimuli needed to make these multiple views? I really don't know. I just know it happens.

Metaphysical Questions Aside

The idea of a moving viewpoint may sound mystical, as if it were some sort of extrasensory perception. This phenomenon could be explained by any number of theories, including the quantum physics concept that perception itself produces effects on the object that is being perceived. Another explanation might be some form of perception that has not yet been identified, like the sonar that gives dolphins a three-dimensional mental image of their surroundings and even allows them to communicate these images to other dolphins. Or it could be conceived as a form of imagination, where the person mentally constructs multiple views of the object or symbol being perceived.

The simple fact is that the mind's eye does perceive multidimensionally, and learning to control its position does allow dyslexics to perceive two-dimensional symbols accurately. Thousands of people have improved their reading and writing skills by learning the techniques described in the following chapters.

If the idea of moving a mental viewpoint around in space sounds far-fetched to you, it's probably because you aren't dyslexic. When I first explain the concept to most dyslexics, they inevitably say, "That's exactly what I do!"

Individuals naturally place their mind's eyes in various advantageous positions. Dancers and athletes (two favorite professions of dyslexics) ordinarily have their mind's eyes positioned above their bodies—a convenient vantage point.

Without getting into theoretical discussions about the nature of reality, let's just say that if a person subliminally causes the mind's eye to rove, he experiences that multidimensional perception as reality.

Finding the Switch

The dyslexic person needs to learn how to turn the disorientation switch on and off. One of the ways to accomplish this is by consciously positioning the mind's eye. When it is moved to a certain place, the person stops being disoriented and is able to perceive the outside or "real" world correctly. The person becomes oriented.

The optimum position of the mind's eye for orientation was discovered through trial and error. It varies with the individual, and can change slightly over time, but it falls within a certain area. The location for orientation is a few inches to a foot above and behind the head, on the centerline of the body. A person who learns to move his mind's eye to what I call his "orientation point" has learned to shut off the distorted perceptions of dyslexia.

The Davis Perceptual Ability Assessment described in the next chapter is used to determine whether a person has the ability to move the mind's eye around easily and see a mental image from different perspectives in space. In other words, can the person intentionally produce disorientation?

The Davis Orientation Counseling Procedure described in chapter 27 is used to teach the person how to control the position of the mind's eye and move it to the optimum viewpoint for real world perception—especially for reading. If the person is not comfortable with intentionally moving the mind's eye, then we can choose a different procedure, called Davis Alignment, to achieve the same result.

The goal of Orientation Counseling or Alignment is not to stop the person from disorienting, for disorientation is a valuable talent. Orientation Counseling or Alignment train the person to turn disorientations on and off at will. With some practice, the mental on-off switch will become available. The person will be able to use it easily.

CHAPTER 25

Implementing the Davis Procedures

This book is *not* intended to be a self-help manual, so a coach or helper is needed. Neither the Orientation Counseling nor the Alignment procedure is designed as a "read-it-and-do-it-to-yourself" exercise, because your attention would be too divided for the process to be effective. You should learn these procedures in order to help someone else to do them, not yourself. If you want to go through one of them yourself, get someone else to read it and practice it, then have him or her guide you through it. That way you can relax and just do it.

The procedures in the following chapter are all the basic methods that have successfully helped dyslexic adults and children since the opening of the Reading Research Council's Dyslexia Correction Center in 1982. In the Davis Orientation Counseling Program, these methods are implemented intensively, five to six hours per day, over the course of five days. Symbol Mastery on the trigger words is started during the program, then completed at home with a parent, spouse or tutor. An intensive schedule has proven best for achieving fast and effective results. A schedule of just one hour a day or one hour per week is effective, but will require more total time because of the loss of momentum between sessions. Just doing "bits and pieces" of the program will fall short of the overall goal of really correcting dyslexia.

A good way to get comfortable with the procedures is to practice them aloud with a friend or act them out by yourself. Go through the explanations and draw the steps on a piece of paper while gathering imaginary answers.

Am I Qualified to Do This?

If you are literate and sincerely want to help someone overcome reading, writing and study problems, the answer is yes. Being willing to spend some time giving a person individual attention and positive feedback is the main credential for using these procedures. Teachers should simply treat these procedures as exercises. They are not harmful. If done wrong, they may produce mild dizziness at worst, which a short walk or nap will relieve. Parents may find these procedures difficult only if they do not first have their child's willingness to participate, or if they use any pressure or coercion.

Small Children vs. Older Dyslexics

The Davis Orientation Counseling and Alignment Procedures are complementary to the Symbol Mastery Procedure. However, they have different objectives. The Davis Orientation Counseling and Alignment Procedures correct perception. Symbol Mastery corrects dyslexia.

Symbol Mastery has also been found to be a useful addition to many curricula for enhancing creativity and language skills. Children under the age of seven or eight (depending on the child's maturity level) are generally better off starting with Symbol Mastery. Younger children can be taught the basic numerals and the alphabet by building them in clay. The basic sight words and reading vocabulary of grades K–2 can be taught using Symbol Mastery for the added benefit of learning their meanings. Children don't have to be dyslexic to use this learning method—it works for all kids. They enjoy it, too!

Later, children who develop dyslexic symptoms can be taught Orientation or Alignment when they are ready—somewhere between age seven (for early developers) and nine (for late developers).

As a general rule, most dyslexics aged eight years or older should start with either the Orientation Counseling or Alignment Procedure, because they are already experiencing the frustration of not being able to read, write or spell well. Part of the gift of dyslexia is the tendency to disorient spontaneously when confused. This way of thinking is on automatic pilot for the dyslexic, and needs to be brought under conscious control. Orientation Counseling or Alignment will enable the person to perceive accurately and consistently when dealing with language and communication.

The Order of the Procedures

Start with the Perceptual Ability Assessment (chapter 26). This will tell you whether to use the Orientation Counseling Procedure or the Alignment Procedure as the tool for terminating disorientations. You should also interview the person to find out what areas of difficulty the person wishes to improve. Even if you think you already know what the person wants help with, it is a good idea to ask anyway. This way the person gets to express it. Parents are often surprised to discover that reading is not at all important to their child, whereas "playing baseball better" or "making friends" is important. By being creative, a parent or teacher can help a child do both better by using the Davis methods.

If the Perceptual Ability Assessment shows that the person can create mental images and move his mind's eye with no problem, the next step is the Davis Orientation Counseling session (chapter 27). If the Perceptual Ability Assessment shows that the person has any difficulty at all with either creating mental images or moving the mind's eye, the appropriate next step is the Alignment Procedure. After the Orientation or Alignment Procedure is complete, follow it with a reading exercise to practice using Orientation or Alignment. This will provide practice right away in detecting and correcting disorientations. Follow this with Dial Setting (chapter 31) to establish and maintain the proper energy levels for different activities. As needed, do Release (chapter 28) to prevent "holding" and headaches.

After the Orientation session, you will be ready to implement the Basic Symbol Mastery steps detailed in chapter 33.

If the Davis Orientation Counseling Procedure is being used, for the next two or three days, do Orientation Review (chapter 28) with the person at the beginning of the day to ensure the orientation point is in the correct place. On the third or fourth day, do Fine Tuning (chapter 29).

After the person has mastered all the basic language symbols (alphabet letters and punctuation marks), proceed to words and begin the Reading Exercises. Once the person is familiar and comfortable with doing Symbol Mastery on some common words (chapter 35), the entire list of Trigger Words should be mastered. This is best done over several months, two to three definitions at a time.

Tips for Symbol Mastery

Treat this procedure as an adventure and a game, not as work. The person should have a desire to improve his or her ability to use written language. You might want to have a discussion about the benefits of being able to read.

Avoid criticizing the artistic qualities of the person's clay creations or correcting them yourself. To encourage accuracy and self-correction, make inquisitive statements like these:

"Check and see if that letter is the same as the example."

"If you weren't going to say anything or use your hands, would the clay say it all?"

"I don't quite see it. Can you show it more clearly?"

"What is it you want to show?"

"Are you satisfied with the way that looks?"

When individuals are first learning the Symbol Mastery techniques, they may not fully get the concept as their own. They may need to repeat the steps on a particular word or concept. But once they are in the groove, mastering a definition once is enough.

Rote repetition or testing the person is not necessary. Once something is done correctly, it's finished. Praise the person and go on to something else. Trust the process to work. The proof will come in the form of increased self-esteem, greater desire to read and progressive improvement in study skills.

You can master the words on the Trigger Word list randomly, in any order, coming back to fill in alternate definitions. One of the gifts of dyslexia is the ability to sort things out automatically. Take advantage of it. Take frequent breaks, just for a few minutes. This lets the knowledge sink in and prevents boredom.

Keep it fun and adventurous. That is the best way to encourage real learning.

CHAPTER 26

Perceptual Ability Assessment

Following is the assessment procedure as taught in the Gift of Dyslexia: Fundamentals of Davis Dyslexia Correction Workshops. It is designed to determine whether a person with a learning disability or other perceptual problem is a candidate for the Orientation Counseling Procedure or the Alignment Procedure. We use this assessment for children and for adults. We do not ordinarily make the assessment on children until the age of seven, because that is when the symptoms of dyslexia typically begin to manifest.

The assessment is arranged in the form of a script, but there is no need to follow any rote procedure once you have a sense of what you are after.

Almost anyone who has the unique perceptual abilities of a dyslexic should be able to do this exercise easily. Pun intended, it should be a piece of cake for them.

However, some dyslexics naturally develop a

kinesthetic or tactile sense that's stronger than their visual sense. As a result they could have some difficulty creating, holding or manipulating mental images. They could also have difficulty shifting their mind's eye. There is also a possibility that an "old solution" could be blocking the picture-making or seeing process (see chapter 5). In addition stress, physical illness and certain medications can also inhibit mental perceptions. For these individuals the Alignment Procedure (see chapter 30) is the orientation procedure that will work for them.

Davis Perceptual Ability Assessment

1. Greeting and Introduction

Greet the person and introduce yourself. As appropriate, explain the nature of the assessment.

2. Concept Clarification

What to Say	What to Do
Are you right handed or left handed?	*Make a note of the answer for future reference.*
What I am interested in is your imagination. Mainly that part of your mind where you can close your eyes and make a picture of something and see the picture. Does that make sense to you?	*If yes, continue. If no, explain further by asking the person, with eyes closed, to imagine something he likes. If the person can't form a mental (imaginary) image, stop.*

143

What to Say	**What to Do**

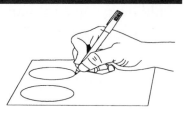

Draw two circles on a blank piece of paper.

This circle represents you.

Point to one of the circles.

This represents me.

Point to the other circle.

If you are looking at me, you are looking *from* here.

Tap your pencil on the first circle.

And you are looking *to* or *at* me over *here*.

Draw an arrow from the first, "you," circle to the second, "me," circle.

As long as we are looking with our eyes, we know exactly where we are looking from. But what about when we are looking at a picture with our minds?

Point at your own eyes.

Pause for a second.

We are doing the same thing. We are looking *at* something— *from* some place.

Point at the "me" circle as you say "at." Point at the "you" circle as you say "from."

I want to call the place we look from the *mind's eye* because it is what sees when we are imagining. It is what is doing the looking.

Make sure they get the idea.

144

What to Say	**What to Do**
Do you like cake?	*Note: Most people like cake, so in this example, we'll assume they do. If "no," try pie, pizza or any distinctly shaped object the person can imagine easily.*
What kind of cake is the best kind?	*Note what kind of cake they like for future reference.*

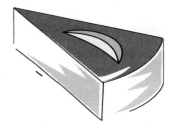

_____

_____

3. Assessment

Have the person sit directly in front of you, close enough that you could reach over and touch his forehead without getting out of your chair, but not so close as to make him feel uncomfortable.

Is it all right if I touch your hands in what we are going to do?

Get their consent.

What to Say

What to Do

We are going to use both of your hands, so I need you to keep them available for me.

Take the person's opposite-to-handedness hand (if he's right-handed, take his left hand; if he's left-handed, take his right). Position the hand, palm up, about where he would hold a book when reading.

Let's imagine a piece of _____ cake is sitting right here in your hand. Tell me when you've got it.

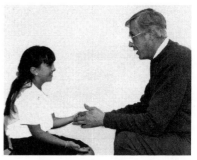

"Imagine a piece of chocolate cake in your hand." (Tap the palm.)

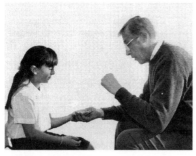

"Close your eyes."

Describe the cake just as he described it, using his exact words: "A big slice of German Chocolate cake," or "Angel food cake with green frosting."

Close your eyes. I want you to keep your eyes closed until I tell you to open them, OK?

Make this request when he says he has a mental picture (if his eyes aren't already closed).

| **What to Say** | **What to Do** |

Note: If the person cannot visualize an object or has difficulty maintaining the image, you can either stop or attempt to coach the person into creating a mental image. Difficulty in visualizing indicates that Orientation Counseling will not be easy for the person and Alignment should be done instead.

By asking simple questions, determine how the imaginary object is positioned in the hand. Continue until you also have a clear mental image of it sitting in the person's hand.

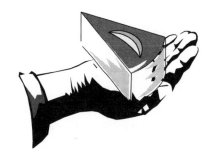

If you cannot make a visual copy of the imaginary object, at least get a sense of its size, shape and position.

Take the index finger of the other hand between your thumb and middle finger. Raise the finger to a point a few inches from the person's forehead, on a level just slightly above eye level.

147

What to Say	What to Do
I want you to shift your imagination and put your mind's eye *here*, where your finger is, and look at the piece of cake from *here*.	
	Tap the tip of his index finger with your index finger as you say "here."
It's as if you raised up a little bit to get another view of the cake from *here*.	*Tap the finger again. Wait several seconds . . .*
Can you see the cake from *here*?	*Tap the finger again.*
	Note: If the person cannot make this first shift easily, do not continue. Go to step 4, ending the assessment. Explain that the assessment is over and that the Alignment Procedure is indicated.

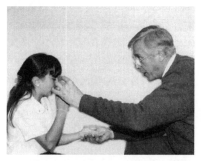

"Look at the piece of cake from here." (Tap the finger.)

I want you to keep your mind's eye in your finger. Now I'm going to move your finger. I want your mind's eye to move with it, OK?	*Note: Do not move the finger while giving instructions or talking to the subject. Make your statement before starting to move the finger and stop moving the finger before you begin talking again.*

148

What to Say	What to Do

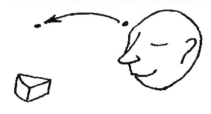

Move the finger slowly and smoothly to a position partway around the open hand. Keep the finger about the same distance from the open hand as the person's eyes are.

Can you see the cake from here?

Tap the finger.

When the person answers yes, ask questions that require a verbal response. Pay attention to response time, variations in speech patterns and any manifestations of confusion or disorientation. Once you are satisfied that the person has actually shifted the mind's eye to the new position, you can go to step 4 and end the assessment at any time.

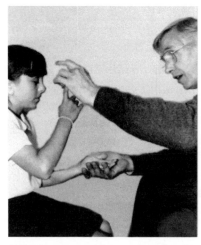

"Can you see the piece of cake from here?"

If you are not sure the person has actually moved the mind's eye, go to the next step.

I am going to move your finger again. I want your mind's eye to move with your finger, OK?

Move the finger slowly and smoothly a little farther around the open hand. Don't move the finger more than a fourth of the distance around, above or below the open hand during any one move.

What to Say	**What to Do**
Can you see the cake from *here*?	*Tap the finger again.*
	When the answer to the question is yes, ask more questions, looking for indications that the person actually has moved the mind's eye. He should see a mental (imaginary) picture from the perspective of his fingertip, as if he were looking at the object from that position.
	Repeat this process of moving the mind's eye and questioning until you are satisfied the mind's eye has actually been moved.

4. Ending the Assessment

I want you to put your mind's eye back in the place where it was when we first started. I want you to get your original view of that piece of cake.	*Slowly and smoothly move the finger toward the eye on the handedness side of the person's body. When within a few inches of the eye, stop the finger.*
Take your mind's eye out of your finger and get your original view of the cake— from your eyes.	*Wait several seconds.*

What to Say	**What to Do**
Do you have your original view?	*When the answer is yes, move the finger in the direction of the lap and release the finger.*
Make the piece of cake go away, and tell me when it is gone.	*Note: If he has any difficulty making the object disappear, have him do a "reverse blink" by rapidly opening and shutting his eyes.*
	When the image is gone, touch the palm of the open hand.
Put another piece of cake here in your hand, and tell me when you have it.	*Note: The reason for forming a second image and making it disappear is to ensure the mind's eye has returned to its original location so the person will not remain disoriented.*
Make this piece of cake go away, and when it is gone, open your eyes.	*When the eyes open, move the open hand toward the lap and release it.*

If the person has any difficulty performing any of the instructions on this assessment, that same difficulty would inhibit him from performing any of the similar steps of the Orientation Counseling Procedure. Therefore, he should not attempt to do the Orientation Counseling. The proper procedure for him is the Alignment Procedure (see chapter 30).

CHAPTER 27

Turning It Around

If the person has dyslexia, the process of correcting it begins with getting the perceptual distortions under control. This means learning how to intentionally turn the disorientations *on* and *off*. The symptoms of dyslexia are the symptoms of disorientation, so once the dyslexic knows how to turn the disorientations off, he can also turn the symptoms off.

Once the disorientations are turned off, the person will stop creating dyslexia symptoms. It may seem that the problem is solved, but orientation is merely the first step of the correction process.

If the Perceptual Ability Assessment indicated the proper orientation procedure is the Davis Orientation Counseling Procedure, use this procedure.

It usually takes less than an hour to put someone through the initial Davis Orientation Counseling session. At the end of a successful session, with some help at catching disorientations as they occur, the dyslexic's reading skill is usually dramatically improved. It can appear that some kind of magic or miracle has just happened, but actually you are only seeing the person's real skills without the interference of disorientations. We have documented cases where the reading ability of teenagers has improved immediately by as many as eight grade levels, as a result of Orientation Counseling alone.

It would be easy to believe something that could produce such a dramatic effect must be difficult to learn. In fact, it is very easy for dyslexics to learn. This is because they already know how to do it. They have been doing it since they were a few months old. They just were not consciously aware of what they were doing all along. Orientation Counseling enables them to understand a skill they already have and gives them a means to control it.

The procedure that follows may sound like a visualization exercise when you read it. Yet when properly applied, it can produce near-miraculous results. There are only a few rules to follow:

1. Make sure the person is a candidate for Orientation Counseling by evaluating his ability to move the mind's eye with the assessment described in the last chapter.
2. Make sure the person wishes to perform the process. He must be willing and eager to do it.

We generally do not perform this process on children younger than seven, because they haven't yet recognized disorientation as a problem at school. As far as they're concerned, nothing needs fixing.

3. Maintain a friendly, supportive control as you guide the person through the steps. He shouldn't have to think about what he's doing, but should simply follow the instructions.

4. Ensure the person is not tired, hungry or taking any medications that interfere with perception or thought.

What follows is a script of an initial Davis Orientation Counseling session as done at the Reading Research Council. Correctly performed, it has produced a 97 percent success rate. If you don't get results, it's likely that one of the four rules listed above has not been followed.

As with the Perceptual Ability Assessment, you are encouraged to use your own words.

Davis Orientation Counseling Initial Session Procedure

1. Greeting and Introduction

Greet the person and establish a rapport. As appropriate, explain the goal and objective of the procedure as stated at the beginning of this chapter.

2. Concept Clarification

If you do not have the notes made during the assessment, you must establish the handedness of the person, and determine an object he can imagine easily. Otherwise, use the same piece of cake or object that was used in the initial assessment.

Explain the concept of orientation as "putting yourself in the proper position in relation to the true facts and conditions of your surroundings."

Explain that disorientation is a condition in which the brain is not receiving what the eyes see or what the ears hear; the balance and movement sense is altered, and the time sense is either speeded up or slowed down.

What to Say	What to Do
Before we start the session, I will go over everything we are going to do. I will show you on paper first, then we'll do it step-by-step. OK?	*Get a piece of paper and have the person sit so the paper can be clearly seen.*

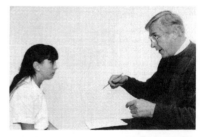

"I'll draw for you exactly what we're going to do so you'll know what to expect."

What to Say	**What to Do**

There are two reasons why we are going over this first. One is to let you know what will be happening so there won't be any surprises. The other is to make sure you understand what I will be asking you to do.

Write on the paper the person's name, your name, the date, the name of the process, the object to be used in visualization and the handedness of the person.

I do ask that you not do any of the process while I'm showing you on the paper. That would only create confusion. Just watch and listen. If you have a question, ask. After we finish going over it on the paper, I will walk you through it step-by-step. OK?

Draw two circles on the paper. Make one circle a top view of a head. Make the other circle a side view of a head.

These are two views of the same head, looking down at it from the top and from the side.

Like in the assessment, we'll have you imagine a piece of _____ in your hand.

Draw the object (the piece of cake used in the assessment) to be visualized in front of both views. On the side view the object should be below eye level, at about a 45-degree angle from the line of sight.

157

What to Say	**What to Do**

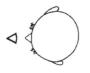

Then we will have you shift your imagination and put your mind's eye in your finger, off to the side, and have you look at the piece of cake from *here*.

Put an X on the person's "handedness" side of the top view to indicate the position of the mind's eye (to the right if the person is right-handed).

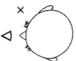

Draw a straight line from the object through the top view. Extend the line well past the back of the head. On the side view, draw a straight line from the object, through the end of the nose, through the head, and extend the line well past the top back of the head.

Once your mind's eye is in your finger, we will have you imagine a line that goes from the piece of cake straight through your head. The line will go from the piece of cake into your nose, through your head, and will stick up about a foot or so above and behind your head.

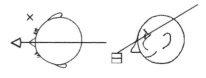

158

What to Say

After you have drawn that line in, we will have you move your mind's eye around so it's a few inches above and behind your head and we'll have you position it on the line. OK?

Do you know how an anchor for a boat works?

You have a heavy weight, and you attach a line or a chain to it. You attach the line to the boat and throw the anchor into the water. The anchor sinks into the mud or hooks on a rock or something, and when the line is pulled tight, the anchor keeps the boat from moving. Right?

We are going to use the same idea as an anchor. When your mind's eye is in the right place on the line above and behind your head, we are going to have you put an anchor line down to the top of each of your ears, and anchor them both in. Then we'll have you put a third anchor line down to the top of your head

What to Do

Make an X on each of the lines going through the heads.

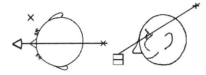

Be sure the concept of "anchor line" is understood.

Draw the three anchor lines on the paper as you explain it.

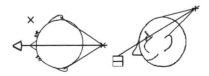

159

What to Say	**What to Do**

and anchor it in there. Then we'll have you pull the three anchor lines straight and attach them together right where your mind's eye is.

Any questions so far?

Once the three anchor lines are drawn in, we won't need the line that goes down to the piece of cake anymore, so you'll erase it out and it will be gone. We won't need the piece of cake anymore either, so we'll have you erase that out also.

To simulate erasing, draw a wavy line over one of the long lines and the object at its end.

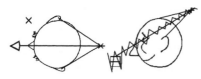

What you will have left are the three anchor lines that come together and make a point above and behind your head.

Draw three lines coming together, separately on another part of the paper. Draw a circle around the intersecting point.

We are going to call the place where the lines come together an orientation point. It is the place where the lines end. We call the lines anchor lines, not to anchor the mind's eye there,

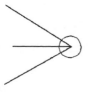

What to Say	What to Do

which you can't do anyway, but to anchor this place there so it is in the same place all the time.

Any questions so far?

What we are really after is a group of brain cells down in the middle of the brain that are responsible for disorientation. When those brain cells are turned *off*, our brain gets exactly what our eyes see, as our eyes are seeing it; and our brain gets exactly what our ears hear, as our ears are hearing it. Our balance and movement sense is accurate, and our sense of time is accurate. When those brain cells are turned *on*, our brain doesn't get what our eyes see; it gets what we think our eyes are seeing. Our brain doesn't get what our ears hear; it gets what we think our ears are hearing. Our balance and movement sense changes, and our internal sense of time can either speed up or slow down.

161

What to Say	**What to Do**

What we really need is the off switch for those brain cells. That's what that orientation point is. It's the off switch for the disorientation.

The way we switch the off switch *off* is simply by putting the mind's eye on that orientation point. That turns those brain cells off.

Draw an X inside the circle where the three separate lines come together.

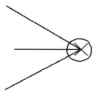

If our mind's eye is sitting in this spot, the brain cells are turned off. But if something happens that can cause a disorientation, the mind's eye doesn't stay there, it moves.

Draw three additional lines coming together, and put an X on the point.

So it takes off, and we are disoriented. In the past, if we waited long enough, or if we went for a walk, or did something other than what we were doing that caused the disorientation, eventually our

Draw an arrow from the point going off to the side.

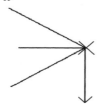

What to Say	What to Do

mind's eye would come back, and we would be all right again—until something else caused another disorientation.

When we have an orientation point, we can deliberately bring the mind's eye back, put it on the point and end the disorientation. We don't have to wait, or do something else, or torture ourselves. Simply putting the mind's eye back in that place turns off the disorientation. It also turns off the feeling of confusion and stops the mistakes.

Draw a line back to the point and retrace the X.

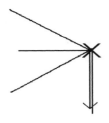

Any questions so far?

Draw three more lines that come together; they should be longer and bolder than the others.

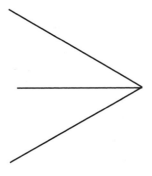

163

What to Say	**What to Do**
Of course, we can't see a mind's eye. In fact, it can't even see itself in a mirror. It is invisible. So we'll just imagine for a moment that this thing is a mind's eye. OK?	
	Pick up some small object (a coin is fine) and hold the object so the person can see it.
When we get to the part of the session where you have put the three anchor lines in, your mind's eye will be sitting right where they come together.	*Position the object on the drawing, right where the three lines come together.*
For the first time in your life, you will have deliberately turned off the brain cells that cause disorientation. The only problem is we don't learn very much from doing something only once.	
So when we have your mind's eye sitting on that point, we are going to find some real-life thing that can cause your mind's eye to jump off the point and disorient you.	*Knock the object off the point where the lines come together.*

What to Say	**What to Do**

When that happens, I'll stop you from looking at the thing that made it jump, and have you simply put your mind's eye back on the point.

Put the object back on the point where the lines come together.

That will turn off the disorientation. The confusion will go away. Then I'll show you what made it happen.

Then we'll find another thing that will make it jump.

Knock the object off the point, and put it back again.

You'll put your mind's eye back, I'll show you what made it jump, and then we'll do it again. We'll do it again and again, until you are an expert at putting your mind's eye back on your orientation point. You will be able to do it quickly, easily and know that you did it.

What you will have then is the ability to turn off a disorientation. It won't matter what turned it on, the action of simply putting your mind's eye on your orientation point will turn it off.

Any questions?

What to Say	**What to Do**

There is one more point we need to make.

We call this a *line*, because it has length to it. Just like this pen/pencil has length to it. But what about when we are looking down the length of it?

Point to one of the anchor lines on the drawing.

Pick up your pen or pencil.

Point the end of the pen/pencil toward the eyes of the person.

It doesn't look long at all, does it? It looks like a dot, doesn't it?

If the mind's eye were sitting right *here*, it wouldn't see the three lines as lines at all, would it?

Point to a place on the drawing where the three lines come together as you say "here."

It would see them as three dots, or as one dot if they were pushed together. Do you agree?

Draw one dot, and also three dots touching each other.

Do you have any questions about what we are going to do?

If you don't have any (more) questions, let's do it!

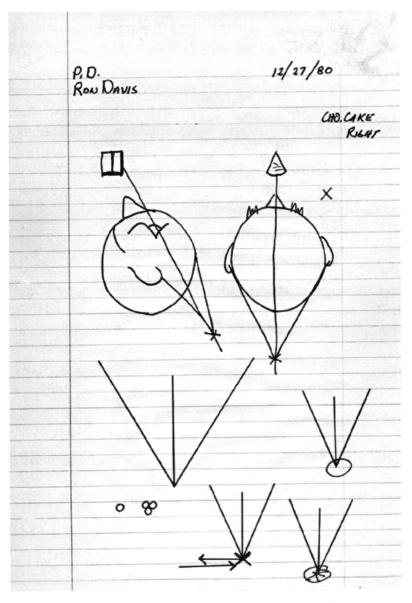

*Your diagram for explaining a Davis Orientation Counseling session
will look something like this when you are finished.*

3. Process Sequence

What to Say	**What to Do**

| | *Have the person sit directly in front of you, close enough that you could reach over and touch his forehead without getting out of your chair. Do not sit so close to the person that you make him feel uncomfortable.* |

Is it all right if I touch your hands in what we're going to do?

Get consent.

We are going to use both of your hands, so I need you to keep them available for me.

Take the person's opposite-to-handedness hand (if he's right-handed, take his left hand; if he's left-handed, take his right). Position the hand, palm up, at the approximate place where a book would be held for reading.

Let's imagine a piece of _____ cake is sitting right here in your hand. Tell me when you've got it.

Describe the cake exactly as it was described to you in the assessment.

Close your eyes *(if not already closed)*. I want you to keep your eyes closed until I tell you to open them, OK?

When you are certain the person has formed a mental image, and his eyes are closed, take the index finger of the other (handedness) hand between your

What to Say	**What to Do**
	thumb and middle finger. Raise the finger to a point off to the side of the forehead on eye level (where you placed the X beside the head on the initial drawing).
I want you to shift your imagination and put your mind's eye *here* . . . where your finger is, and look at the piece of cake from *here*.	*Tap the index finger with your index finger as you say "here."*
It's the same as if you leaned over and are looking from *here*.	*Tap the finger again. Wait several seconds.*
Can you see the piece of cake from *here*?	*Tap the finger. When yes, go to the next step.*
Imagine a straight line that goes from the piece of cake into your nose, through your head, and sticks up about a foot behind you. Draw that line in, and tell me when you have it there.	*Confirm that the line is there.*
I am going to move your finger. I want your mind's eye to move with it, OK?	*Note: Do not move the finger while giving instructions or talking to the person. Finish making your statement before starting to move the finger and stop moving the finger before you begin talking again.*

What to Say	**What to Do**
I want to put your mind's eye on the line above and behind your head, so let me move your finger. Let your mind's eye move with it.	*You will need to stand up to reach above and behind the person's head. Do so quietly and gently.*

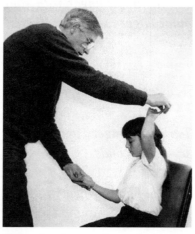

Stop the finger 6 to 10 inches above and behind the head.

	Move the finger <u>slowly</u> and <u>smoothly</u> toward the midline of the body above and behind the head. Stop the finger about 6 to 10 inches above and behind the head.
	If the person's elbow is sticking out to the side of his body, you may need to turn his shoulder so the elbow points forward. This way the hand can easily reach behind the head.
I can't see the line. Only you can see it, so I need you to make the fine adjustment to get the mind's eye right on it.	*Loosen your grip on the index finger and allow the person to move the finger freely. It may take several seconds for the person to find the exact spot. When the person stops moving the finger, grasp it again.*

What to Say	**What to Do**

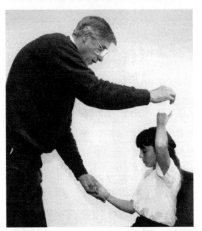

"*I'll need you to make the final adjustment to get your mind's eye right on the line.*"

[It seems to be a bit off to the side. Is it all right if I move it just a bit?]

Pull the line to come to here and tell me when you've got it.

Look to see that the finger is on what would be the midline of the body (it seldom is).

If it is on midline, go to the next step.

[If it is not on the midline, without changing the distance from the head, move the finger to the midline.]

Tap the finger.

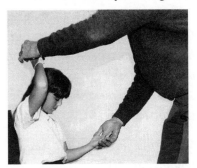

"*Pull the line to here.*" (*Move the finger to the midline and tap it.*)

171

What to Say	**What to Do**
Can you see your ears from *here*? You can see right through your hair.	
	Tap the finger.
	When yes, go to the next step.
	[If no, have the person "feel" where the ears would be. If necessary, have him feel his ears with his hand (use the hand holding the imaginary object). If feeling them does not bring about seeing them, have the person imagine where his ears would be and make a
Put anchor lines down to the top of each ear, anchor them in, and pull them straight to *here*.	*mental picture of them.]*
	Tap the finger.
Put another anchor line down to the top of your head, anchor it in and pull it straight to *here*, as well.	
	Tap the finger.
Attach the three lines together.	*Confirm that the three anchor lines have been attached*
I want to move your finger, but I don't want your mind's eye to come with it this time. OK?	*together.*
	Get agreement.
As I move your finger, leave your mind's eye at the end of the lines.	*Move the finger to the side a few inches.*

172

What to Say	**What to Do**
Did your mind's eye stay on the lines?	*If yes, move the finger over the shoulder in the direction of the lap. Release the finger and sit back down.* *[If no, take the finger back to the position on the lines.]*
[Take your mind's eye out of your finger and leave it on the lines when I move your finger.]	*[Repeat this step until the mind's eye remains on the lines.]*
We don't need the line that goes down to the piece of cake anymore, so erase it out and tell me when it is gone. We also don't need the piece of cake anymore, so erase it out and tell me when it is gone.	
What color are the three anchor lines you just put in?	*Make a note about the color choice for your reference.*
Move your mind's eye to the place where the three (color) lines come together. Tell me when it is there.	
Do you see three dots or one?	*Make a note about the number of dots.*

173

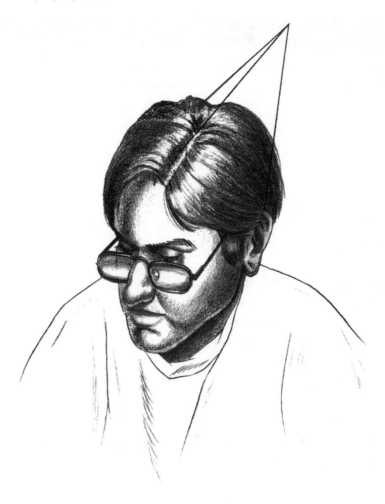

The anchor lines put in by the dyslexic during Davis Orientation Counseling will converge at a point six to ten inches above and behind the head. It will be at approximately a 45-degree angle, precisely on the midline of the body.

What to Say	**What to Do**
Are the dots the same color as the lines?	*Make a note about the color of the dots.*

What your mind's eye sees right now is what it should see when it is on the orientation point. Anytime you want to, you can look with your mind's eye. If it sees what it sees right now, you know it is on the orientation point.

If it doesn't see what it sees right now, you would know that it isn't on the orientation point and you would have to move it to the point to see what it sees now. Any questions?

Open your eyes. Did it move when you opened your eyes?	*If no, go to the next step.*
	[If yes, tell him to put it back.]
[Put it back.]	
[Close your eyes and look.]	*[If "I don't know," have him close his eyes and check.]*

175

4. Explanation

What to Say	What to Do

I can't see your mind's eye. I can't see your anchor lines. If I hadn't been here while you were doing this, I wouldn't even know that you have them. If I can't tell, nobody else can tell either, so only you know for sure. You don't have to be concerned that anybody will think you are weird or that you are doing something that they can't do.

You can't touch a mind's eye; nothing can.

You don't have to worry about anything hitting it; or knocking it into a wall, a door or anything else. You don't have to worry about catching it in the car door. It goes right through things, like they aren't even there.

When your mind's eye is sitting on the point, it is located by the lines that go to your ears and the top of your head. You can't move fast enough to lose it.

Wave your hand above and behind your head.

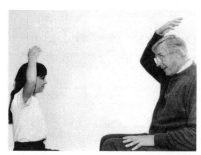

"You don't have to worry about knocking your mind's eye off or anyone seeing your lines."

What to Say	**What to Do**

You can't turn your head fast enough to knock it off. It just sits there and goes where your head and ears go.

Any questions?

Do you know what the word *responsibility* means?

Whether the answer to the question is yes or no, get the concept of responsibility across.

Let me give you a simple/ simpler definition. Responsibility is the ability and the willingness to control something. Control in its simplest form is the ability to cause something to change, or to cause it not to change.

Because I can reach over and move your hand, I am changing something about your body. That change is happening, and you're not doing it. I am responsible for that change. You aren't, because you didn't do it. Right?

Take one of the person's hands and move it a bit.

But I can't reach over and move your mind's eye. No one can. There isn't a person, animal,

What to Say	What to Do

machine or anything on this earth that can move your mind's eye one-billionth of an inch. But you can put it anywhere you want to. That means that you have total control, which also means that you have total responsibility for where your mind's eye is and what it does.

Do you agree?

That also means that when it jumps, when you get disoriented, you are the one that made it jump. When you were very young, you set it up so that whenever you were confused enough, your mind's eye would automatically go off and try to get rid of the confusion. When the confusion was about a real object, that actually worked. It would get rid of the confusion. But it won't work with a symbol, and all words are symbols, so it won't work with words. Moving the mind's eye around just creates more confusion.

178

What to Say

What to Do

Now you have a problem. Your mind's eye jumps every time you get confused, and you don't want it to do that anymore.

The problem is, it is still going to jump. If you try to hold it on the point to keep it from jumping, while at the same time you are automatically trying to make it jump, you are going to get a headache.

The only solution I know is to go ahead and let it jump. When it does, simply bring it back. That will be your job, your responsibility. Whenever it jumps, you put it back.

Do you have any questions?

Is your mind's eye still sitting on your orientation point?

If yes, go to the next step.

[Put it back on the point.]

[If no, have the person put it back.]

For the first little while after we get an orientation point, our mind's eye just floats around it.

179

What to Say	What to Do

It doesn't just sit there. This happens to everyone. We call it "drifting."

As soon as you get used to controlling your mind's eye, putting it and leaving it on the orientation point, the drifting will stop. Then when you put your mind's eye there it will just sit there.

Don't try to hold your mind's eye there, just let it drift. Every once in a while, move it back to the point and let go of it. If you try to hold it there, you are just prolonging the drifting phase.

Any questions?

5. Practicing Using Orientation

Based on the person's disorientation history, select an activity, such as reading, that will disorient him. Be alert for indications of disorientation. When a disorientation or mistake occurs, stop the activity.

What to Say	**What to Do**
Did your mind's eye move?	*If the answer is no, continue the activity until it does.*
	[If "I don't know," have him check.]
[Look with your mind's eye and see if it sees the dot/dots.]	
	When the mind's eye has moved, have the person put it back.
Put it back.	*Then point out the stimulus that triggered the disorientation.*

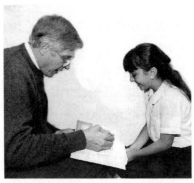

Point out each word that triggers a disorientation.

Continue in this fashion until the person can quickly and easily put the mind's eye back on the orientation point, and sees that it makes a difference.

When the person can quickly and easily put the mind's eye on the orientation point, and knows that he has done so, the session is complete.

181

CHAPTER 28

Release and Orientation Review

As the dyslexics using the Davis Orientation Procedure develop orientation skills, it will become obvious to them that *if the mind's eye doesn't move, there are no mistakes.* As they become more aware of their state of orientation, they will notice that whenever their mind's eye moves, they disorient. After they disorient, either they will make a reading mistake or some "old solution" will automatically turn on.

It would seem that the next logical skill to develop would be a method of keeping the mind's eye on the orientation point. It is simple to do, and most individuals will try it. Unfortunately, this usually results in an intense headache.

The probable reason is that the mind's eye doesn't really move by itself. The person is, on a subconscious level, causing it to move. Moving it is an ingrained habit. Learning about orientation and the benefits of not moving the mind's eye won't prevent the person from having this natural reaction to confusion.

So when the person becomes confused, he will be attempting to move the mind's eye at the same time he is trying to prevent it from moving—literally working against himself. We call this *holding.* It creates tension, which results in the headache.

Simply telling the person not to hold their mind's eye on the orientation point does not work. It's like telling them not to think about an elephant: It will cause them to do it instead of preventing it. The more they try not to hold, the stronger the holding will become.

Anyway, there is no reason not to disorient when it's appropriate and useful.

Individuals who are holding the mind's eye rigidly on the orientation point will usually reach up and rub the back of their neck. When you see them do this, intervene with the Release Procedure.

Signs of Holding
1. The person complains of a headache.
2. The person rubs or touches the back of the neck.
3. The skin tone becomes pale.
4. The brows wrinkle.
5. The person begins to look stressed or distressed.

The Release Procedure can be used for conditions other than holding. It is very effective in eliminating the stress and tension that result from engaging in intense activities of any kind. As such, the procedure should be done with Alignment Procedure users as well.

Release Procedure

Have individuals go through the Release Procedure by reading or reciting these steps to them. As you go, make sure they perform the action requested before doing the next step. If they say they "can't," or aren't certain whether they have done a step, say, "Imagine what it would be like to do that."

Make a loose fist—not too tight. Just let your fingers curl into your palm. Now think the thought "open hand," but instead of opening your hand, make the fist tighter.

Think the thought again, "open hand," and make the fist even tighter.

Again think the thought "open hand," and make the fist really tight—really, *really* tight, tight all the way up to your elbow.

Now without thought simply let your hand release. Let your entire hand go. Let your fingers find their natural place.

Feel the feeling that goes down your arm, through your hand, all the way out to the tips of your fingers. That feeling is the feeling of *release.* When the word *release* is used, that feeling is what is meant.

The feeling of release is also the same feeling as the feeling of a sigh.

Do a sigh. Breathe in and hold it for a second or two. Then let the air rush out your mouth, with a "hunnnn" sound coming from your nose and throat.

A little sigh puts the feeling of release in your upper chest. A great big sigh can put that feeling all the way out to the tips of your fingers and toes.

Do a great big sigh. Get that feeling all through your body. Now let that feeling linger. Let that feeling remain in your body.

Now let your mind's eye have that feeling, by simply wanting it to. Your mind's eye can have that feeling. That's what your mind's eye should feel like.

Now have your mind's eye put that feeling down into your head and neck. You'll feel your neck muscles letting go. You'll feel them get loose.

If the person has a headache, use this step before continuing:

Now have your mind's eye put that feeling right inside the headache. Have your mind's eye fill up the headache with the feeling of release.

Have your mind's eye continue filling up the headache with release until it is completely gone.

In the future, whenever you have to put your mind's eye back on the orientation point, after you've got it there, let it go. Turn loose of it. It won't go anywhere, it'll just sit there. You don't have to hold it.

Every time you have to bring your mind's eye back, let it have that feeling of release. Then you won't have the headaches or the old solutions happening anymore.

After the person has learned what Release is and how to do it, there is no need to go through the whole procedure again. Simply ask or remind the person to "do Release" whenever you notice him holding, concentrating, tensing up or exerting a lot of effort.

Orientation Review Procedure

After a few hours, the orientation point established in the initial Orientation Counseling session may change location. As a result, from time to time you may need to check and see if it has moved and, if so, put it back to its original place. This is done with the Orientation Review Procedure.

Simply ask the person to put their finger where their orientation point is. Typically when I do it, I say: "Earlier when we did the orientation session, you got something called an orientation point. It's the place where the three lines make the point. Can you put your finger where that point is?"

When they do, check to see that their finger is on the midline of their body and between six and ten inches above and behind the head. If they put their finger in the right place, say: "That's good. Keep using that point and everything should be just fine."

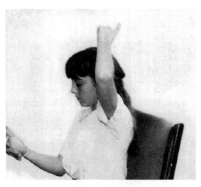

The right place.

187

If they put their finger anywhere other than in the right place, simply ask if you can do a "slight adjustment." (No one has ever said no.)

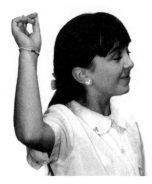

Her mind's eye is too low and off to the right.

Grasp their finger between your thumb and middle finger, and gently pull it to the midline of the body. Tap the end of their finger with your index finger and say: "Pull the point to here by adjusting the lines. Tell me when you've got it here." Tap the finger again.

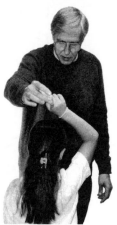

Adjust the point and lines to the midline.

188

When they tell you that the point is now where you want it, tell them: "That's good. Use this point, and everything should be just fine."

If the point continues to shift excessively after doing the above adjustment, tell the person to "set the lines so they won't move."

Use Orientation Review only until you do the Fine Tuning Procedure covered in the next chapter. After doing Fine Tuning, this method of checking the location of the orientation point is no longer appropriate.

CHAPTER 29

Fine Tuning

The Fine Tuning Procedure is a method for the oriented dyslexic to find his or her *optimum orientation point.* It is named for the process used to fine-tune a radio by moving the knob back and forth until the best possible reception is found.

The same thing can be done with the mind's eye. By moving it around the existing orientation point, the optimum place for orientation can be located.

There are several things to keep in mind here. The Fine Tuning Procedure is best done after the oriented dyslexic has had at least two days' experience at controlling orientation. Fine Tuning should not be attempted until any and all drifting (slight floating of the mind's eye) has stopped.

During Fine Tuning the mind's eye can move in every direction, not just back and forth. Also, at any time the mind's eye is moving, a person will feel out of balance. Fine Tuning is done by moving it just a little, stopping it and checking how things feel.

There are two ways a person can tell when they have reached their optimum orientation place. First, they will be perfectly balanced. They can stand on one foot without any movement in their foot, ankle, knee, hips or torso. They can hold that position until their muscles become physically tired. At that point, they can still remain comfortably balanced by simply switching to the other foot. Secondly, when their mind's eye is at their optimum orientation place, the individual will experience a profound feeling of well-being—what I call the *comfort zone*. It will just "feel right."

Often while doing Fine Tuning, the person will move their mind's eye through the comfort zone. When this happens, the feeling of well-being will "wash" over them momentarily. They will probably smile, and will look relieved. But if they don't stop their mind's eye at that exact location, the feeling will vanish as quickly as it occurred.

Assuming we start with the mind's eye above and behind the head, the observable phenomena of the relationship between the mind's eye and the body are:

1. If the mind's eye is left of midline, the body is out of balance to the left.
2. If the mind's eye is right of midline, the body is out of balance to the right.

191

3. If the mind's eye is too far back, even if on the midline, the body is out of balance in the backward direction.
4. If the mind's eye is too far forward, even if on the midline, the body is out of balance in the forward direction.
5. If the mind's eye is too low, the body is out of balance in the backward direction.
6. If the mind's eye is too high, the body is out of balance in the forward direction.
7. If the mind's eye is in front of the centerline of the body, (1) and (2) above reverse.

Using the above information, the person can find the optimum orientation point.

The person does the procedure by slowly moving and stopping the mind's eye within the general area of the existing orientation point. This is done until perfect balance is achieved, and he or she experiences an overall feeling of well-being.

Fine Tuning Procedure

As in all these procedures, use your own words.

What to Say	**What to Do**

Explain the concept of fine-tuning a radio and how it can apply to finding optimum orientation.

I want you to keep your eyes open during what we're about to do, OK?

Find a location where there is a view that extends a long way. This can be looking out of a window. Have the person stand facing the view.

Put your mind's eye on your orientation point.

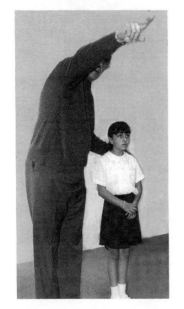

Have the person check to see that the mind's eye is on the orientation point.

Stand next to the person and point out a particular spot or point in the vista. The spot or point should not be below eye level.

"Look at that picture up there."

What to Say	**What to Do**

With your eyes looking at that spot/point, balance on one foot.

Note: It does not matter which foot the person balances on. He can switch feet if he wishes.

Gently grasp the person by the shoulders, then release the grasp without moving your hands far from the shoulders.

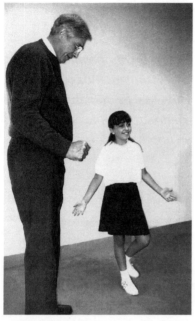

"Keep looking at it and balance on one foot."

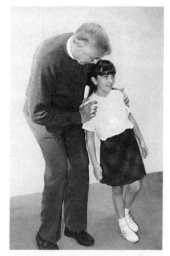

"Give it a push and see what happens."

Now push your mind's eye off your point in my direction, and see what it does to your balance. I won't let you fall.

[Give it a good push; I won't let you fall.]

If the person doesn't lean into you . . .

What to Say	**What to Do**

Put your mind's eye back on point and put your foot down.

Note: It is important that the person feels the body go out of balance in the direction the mind's eye moves.

Locate another spot or point that is closer, about 45 degrees below the line of sight. Direct the person's attention to the spot/point.

Tip your head forward and look directly at the spot/point. Now balance on one foot.

Now, just like fine-tuning a radio, move your mind's eye around and find the place where your body is in perfect balance.

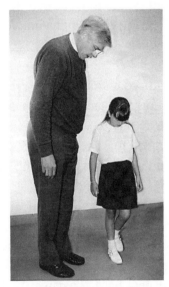

Remember, while your mind's eye is moving, your balance is out, so move it just a bit, stop it, and then check. You'll know when you've got it by the feeling that it has.

"Look at that dime I threw on the floor and balance on one foot."

Note: This process takes as long as it takes. The person may not find optimum orientation on the first attempt.

What to Say	What to Do

Don't let the person stop unless he is very close to, or has actually found, the optimum orientation place.

When the person has found optimum orientation, or is getting tired and is very close, use the following steps to end the process.

Hold your mind's eye right where it is, and put your foot down.

Hold your mind's eye right where it is, and pull your dot/ dots to where your mind's eye is. You're not moving the mind's eye; you're moving the point *to* the mind's eye.

Let your anchor lines set up and get hard right where they are, just like concrete sets up and gets hard. That way your point will be right where it should be and won't be moving around.

Confirm that this has been done.

Explain that the person should use this procedure at least once a day to make sure the orientation point is optimum. Explain that, from time to time, the optimum place changes location for reasons unknown, and the person must adapt to that change using this procedure.

After Fine Tuning, do not have the person try to put their finger where the point is. They probably won't be able to find it, and asking them to do so will only create confusion.

Future Orientation Review is done by simply having the person look down and balance on one foot, showing you that the balance is there.

There is only one optimum orientation point where all sensory data is most accurate. However, there are other orientation locations, one or more for each of the senses, where that sense will be very acute. The one for balance is two feet or more directly above the head, or forward of the center of gravity. When working with athletes, dancers and so on (anyone with excellent balance), make sure they are orienting above and behind the head and not directly above or in front of it. Having the person look down while checking should ensure this.

CHAPTER 30

Alignment Procedure

The Davis Alignment Procedure is the beginning step in the Davis Dyslexia Correction process for some dyslexics. If the person you are working with had any difficulty performing any of the steps in the Perceptual Ability Assessment, this is the procedure to use.

Just like the Davis Orientation Counseling Procedure, this procedure will enable the person to intentionally turn the disorientations on and off. The symptoms of dyslexia are the symptoms of disorientation, so once the dyslexic knows how to turn the disorientations off, he can also turn the symptoms off.

Once the disorientations are turned off, the person will stop creating dyslexia symptoms. It may seem that the problem is solved, but orientation is merely the first step of the correction process.

When using Alignment, the Alignment Fine Tuning Procedure and Koosh Ball Exercises (chapter 32) can follow immediately. This gives the person these additional tools right away. This is especially helpful when there are significant issues with dyspraxia and coordination.

When doing the Alignment Procedure for the first time with someone, you will be doing three separate procedures as if they were only one. Always start this process by doing the Release Procedure first. Then do the Alignment Procedure, and immediately follow with the Alignment Fine Tuning Procedure. These three procedures are laid out here in the sequence to be followed, so that when guiding someone through it, you can simply read the script aloud.

First, however, you must set the stage. You must prepare the person for what will be coming and what to expect. As with the Davis Orientation Counseling Procedure, prepare an explanation of why you are giving the person this tool. Tailor the explanation to the individual. Use words that will be understood. Keep in mind that you are talking to someone who probably isn't very good at thinking with words. Keep the explanation as short and specific as possible.

In addition, the person to whom you are giving the explanation may have a very short attention span. If you talk longer than his attention span, you will lose him. Sometimes this can happen in as little as five to ten seconds. Any explanation you give will take longer than that, so use a strategy to get you beyond that limit. Break the explanation up. Talk for a few seconds and then ask the person to respond in some way. For the most part, asking questions that require only a yes or no answer will suffice.

There isn't a set script to follow, so you will have to play it by ear. Here is an example of what one might ask and say to a seven-year-old child:

> *What we're about to do is called Alignment. Have you ever heard that word before?*
>
> *It's a name for a tool that can help you focus and do better in school.*
>
> *Do you think it would be good to have a tool that would help you make fewer mistakes?*

Only if the answer to the last question is yes would you continue. If the answer is no, you may have a motivation problem, or the person didn't really understand your explanation.

When guiding someone through the initial Alignment session, you can read aloud the following script. Continue to use short segments to address short attention span; responses can now be nonverbal, such as a nod of the head.

Release

Get comfortable—as comfortable as you can.

Make a loose fist—not too tight. Just let your fingers curl into your palm.

Now think the thought "open hand," and make the fist tighter. Think the thought again, "open hand," and make the fist even tighter.

Again, think the thought "open hand," and make the fist really tight—tight all the way up to your elbow.

Now without thought, simply let your hand go; let your fingers find their natural place.

Feel the feeling that goes down your arm, through your hand, all the way out to the tips of your fingers. That feeling is the feeling of release. When the word *release* is used that feeling is what is meant.

The feeling of release is the same feeling as the feeling of a sigh.

Do a sigh. Breathe in, hold it for a second, now let the air rush out of your mouth, with the "hunnnn" sound coming from your throat and chest.

A little sigh puts the feeling of release in your upper chest. A great big sigh can put that feeling all the way out to the tips of your fingers and toes. Do a great big sigh; get that feeling all through your body. Now let that feeling linger; let that feeling remain in your body.

Close your eyes. Feel your toes; find where your toes are and feel them from the inside.

Hold your feeling of your toes and feel your fingers. Find where your fingers are and feel them from the inside.

Now expand your feeling from your toes all the way to your ankles and from your fingers all the way to your wrists.

Now continue to expand your feeling from your toes all the way to your knees, and from your fingers all the way to your elbows.

Continue all the way to your hips and shoulders.

Now all through your body, all the way up to your neck.

Now all through your neck and head, all the way to the skin on top of your head. Get it all, including your ears.

Now do a great big sigh and flood your entire body with the feeling of release, all the way out to the tips of your fingers and toes.

Let that feeling of release remain in your body, and when it is comfortable to do so, allow your eyes to open.

Alignment

Close your eyes again. The feeling of Release should still be in your body.

Without moving your body, get the feeling that you are getting up. Get the feeling that you are getting up out of your chair.

Now get the feeling that you are moving around and standing behind the body.

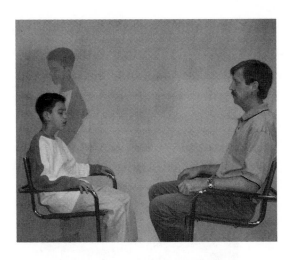

Have the feeling that you are standing right behind the body that is sitting in front of you.

Reach out and put your imaginary hands on the shoulders of the body sitting in front of you.

Feel your shoulders with your imaginary hands, and feel your imaginary hands with your real shoulders.

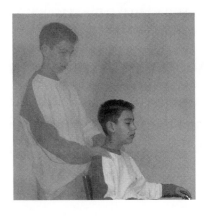

Open your imaginary eyes and look down on the body sitting in front of you. You should see the top and back of the head.

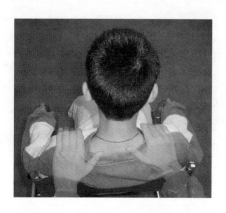

Close your imaginary eyes and keep the feeling of your imaginary hands on your shoulders.

Open your eyes. Keeping the feeling of the hands on the shoulders, look around the room. Look at the things in relation to where your body is. See where the walls are in relation to your body.

(Allow the person to make observations and comments.)

Alignment Fine Tuning

Stand up, keeping the imaginary hands on your shoulders. Stand clear of the table and any chairs. Balance on one foot. Let the imaginary hands hold you in balance.

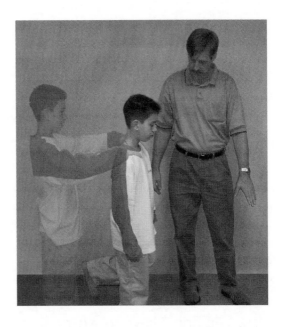

If you feel out of balance in any direction, move the imaginary body slightly in the opposite direction until you feel in perfect balance.

When you have found your perfect balance, lock your imaginary elbows, so the imaginary body will always be in the same position when the imaginary hands are on your shoulders.

Now you can walk around, keeping the imaginary hands on your shoulders.

Anytime you want to or need to, you can realign by getting the feeling of having your imaginary hands on your shoulders.

Explanation

The following script should be conducted as a conversation, not read aloud as the previous steps:

I can't see your imaginary hands. If I hadn't been here while you were doing this, I wouldn't even know that you have them.

If I can't tell, nobody else can tell either, so only you know for sure. You don't have to be concerned that anybody will think you are weird or that you are doing something that they can't do.

You don't have to worry about anything hitting the imaginary body or knocking it into a wall, a door or anything else. You don't have to worry about catching it in the car door. It goes right through things, like they aren't even there.

You can't turn fast enough to knock it away. It is just there when you want it by feeling the imaginary hands. Any questions?

Do you know what the word *responsibility* means?

Let me give you a simple/simpler definition.

Responsibility is the ability and the willingness to control something. Control in its simplest form is the ability to cause something to change, or to cause it not to change.

Because I can reach over and move your hand, I am changing something about your body. That change is happening, and you're not doing it. I am responsible for that change; you aren't, because you didn't do it. Right?

But I can't reach over and move your imaginary hands. No one can. There isn't a person, animal, machine or anything on this earth that can move your imaginary hands one-billionth of an inch. But you can put them anywhere you want to. That means that you have total control, which also means that you have total responsibility for where your imaginary hands are and what they do. Do you agree?

That also means that when you get disoriented and your imaginary hands leave, you are the one that made them leave. This is because when you were very young, you set it up so that whenever you were confused enough, your imagination would automatically go off and try to get rid of the confusion. When the confusion was about a real object, it actually worked; it would get rid of the confusion. But it won't work with a symbol, and all words are symbols, so it won't work with words. It just creates more confusion.

Now when you get or feel confused, just feel the imaginary hands on your shoulders. That will stop the problem. So it will be your job, your responsibility, whenever they leave, for you bring them back. Do you have any questions?

Are your hands still on your shoulders? (If no, say: "Feel the imaginary hands on your real shoulders.")

Practice Using Alignment

Based on the disorientation history, select an activity, such as reading, that will disorient the person. Be alert for indications of disorientation. When a disorientation or mistake occurs, stop the activity and ask, "Did your imaginary hands move?"

If the answer is no, continue the activity until they do.

If the answer is "I don't know," have the person feel his imaginary hands on his real shoulders to check, then continue the activity until the answer is yes.

If or when the answer is yes, say, "Put them back on your shoulders."

Point out the stimulus that triggered the disorientation, and continue with the activity. Continue until the person can quickly and easily feel his imaginary hands on his shoulders, and can see that it makes a difference.

When the person can quickly and easily feel his imaginary hands on his shoulders, the session is complete.

Alignment Review Procedure

For those individuals using Alignment the Review Procedure is very simple. Have the person get the feeling of the imaginary hands on the shoulders and balance on one foot; first one then the other. If the balance is right on, nothing needs be done. However, if the balance is off, instruct the person to release the locked elbows and adjust the location of the imaginary body to bring about balance. When the balance is right on, instruct the person to lock the elbows so the balance won't change.

A NOTE OF CAUTION: *The product of both the Davis Orientation Counseling Procedure and the Alignment Procedure is accurate perception. Either procedure is capable of producing that product. However, if an attempt is made to use both procedures at the same time, there may be unpredictable distortions in the person's perception. If this happens, it can be difficult to undo, and the person may be left with an aversion to using either tool. Therefore, use one of the procedures or the other, but not both.*

CHAPTER 31

Dial Setting

With disorientation, there is distortion in perception and variations in brain chemistry that affect a person's experience of time and energy. The variations in brain chemistry explain many of the symptoms and characteristics of attention deficit disorder, including hyperactivity (high energy, internal time is racing) or hypoactivity (low energy, internal time is crawling).

With orientation, there is accuracy in perception and a stabilizing effect in the brain chemistry. Once a person has control of his or her orientation, control over the experience of time and energy levels can be established by setting up an "energy dial."

Even though this procedure was originally developed for controlling hyperactivity or restlessness, we now recommend it for anyone using the procedures in this book. Having an energy dial gives a person control over the experience of time and energy, such as feeling rushed, bored or sleepless. It can also enhance performance in many other aspects of life, such as athletics, social interactions and communications.

A dial, according to the dictionary, is a circle around or on which a scale is marked, with a pointer that rotates around the center of the circle. A dial does two things: first, it is a gauge that shows the functioning level of something and second, it is or can be the control for altering or changing some function or functions. A common example is the control for a stove burner.

For our purposes, we want the dial to control the rate at which the person experiences change (time or speed), and the energy level the person is experiencing.

We create the dial using imagination and feeling. We want the person to be oriented or aligned before we start this, because the person's intention will then be stronger, and the perceptions more accurate.

Dial Setting can be done anytime after the Orientation Counseling session or Alignment/Fine Tuning session. It is always preceded by the Release Procedure (see Chapter 28).

The Dial Setting Procedure

After having the person do the Release Procedure, ask if he or she knows what a dial is. Explain it if the person doesn't know. Make sure the person understands that a dial shows the level of a function and that it controls the level of that function.

Ask the person to imagine a dial that shows his or her energy level. Have the person describe it. It is best if the dial has ten graduations on it, so if what is described does not, ask the person to change the image so that there are ten graduations on it, from 1 to 10.

Have the person position the dial somewhere in front, to the left or right side, but not directly in front. To ensure this has occurred, have the person put a hand in the space where the image of the dial is.

Ask him, "If the dial shows your energy level right now, where is the dial set?"

If it is 5 or below, have the person set the dial up two or three notches (to at least 7). Ask the person, "Do you feel the surge of energy? Do you feel the change in temperature in your body? Do you notice the feeling of being more awake? Do you feel jittery at this level?"

If it is above 5, have the person set the dial down two or three notches (to at least 3). Ask the person, "Do you feel yourself slowing down? Do you feel the calming feeling? Do you feel the cooling feeling? Do you feel the relaxing feeling?"

There may be other questions you want to ask that would be appropriate for the particular person. Ask the questions to draw the person's attention to the physical changes he experiences. Do not question whether the person's answer is correct or not. Do not make the person feel wrong for what he notices.

When the person notices the differences, ask him to set the dial in the *opposite direction*, two or three notches below or above the original setting, and ask the questions listed above appropriate to the setting change. When the person notices the differences, have him set the dial at its original setting and notice the changes there. Because the change is less, the difference in feelings will be more subtle; however, the person will be able to feel it.

After the dial is created and established, you can discuss with the person the "appropriate dial settings" for various activities. Also, in the future you can ask the person where his dial is set at and he will be able to tell you. For a while you may need to remind the person of the appropriate dial settings, until he begins automatically adjusting the dial in relation to what he is doing. Keep in mind that dial settings are individual; one person's 5 may be another's 8 and vice versa. Allow each person to determine (and experiment with and change) the appropriate dial settings for various activities.

CHAPTER 32

Coordination

After the Fine Tuning process is completed, there is a fast and simple way to put an end to *left/right confusion* problems for good. This process also addresses the dyspraxia problem described in chapter 11. We call it Koosh Ball Therapy because we use the light, furry toy balls made of rubber band material for the process. We don't recommend other balls like tennis balls or Ping-Pong balls, because they have a tendency to bounce out of people's hands before they're able to grasp them.

You can start doing this therapy periodically after the Fine Tuning Procedure is completed.

Stand six to ten feet away from the person (closer for small children). Start by telling the person to "check your point." When the person is on point (oriented or aligned), have him balance on one foot. He should be able to stand on either foot, and switch feet at any time.

Hold both balls in one hand. When the person is

comfortably balanced on one foot, say, "Catch one ball in one hand and the other ball in the other hand."

1. Underhanded, toss each ball, one at a time. Toss gently, aiming about chest high. Each time you toss a ball, say, "One in one hand, one in the other."
2. When the person can easily catch a ball in either hand without losing balance, repeat, "One in one hand, one in the other." Then toss both balls *simultaneously*. Aim for a position directly in front of the person, on the midline of the body. If the balls are properly tossed, one ball will be on each side of the midline. Be sure to toss them so they can be easily caught.

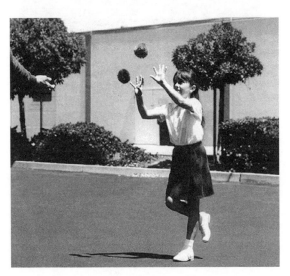

"One in one hand, one in the other."

215

When the person catches both balls, praise him and do it again.

3. After a while, say, "I am going to toss them both to one side of you. I want you to catch them without losing your balance." Do this for each side so the person has to cross the midline with the opposite hand to catch both balls. Don't aim too far to the side, or you will cause the person to lose balance.

This exercise makes a good break activity while doing Symbol Mastery on the Trigger Words (see chapter 35).

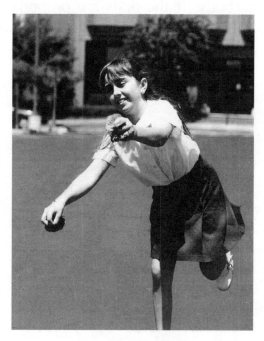

Crossing the midline.

CHAPTER 33

Basic Symbol Mastery

Earlier, I mentioned that confusion about the meanings of trigger words was the underlying cause of the disorientations that cause the symptoms of dyslexia. The Trigger Words are the most important culprits, but there are many other symbols that can cause disorientations as well. Most dyslexics will "trigger" on some individual letters of the alphabet and on some punctuation marks. Some will also trigger on some speech sounds, math symbols and numbers.

To truly correct the learning disability of dyslexia, all the triggering words and symbols must be learned so thoroughly that they are mastered.

Ideally, these exercises should be done individually with the student, at the student's pace. Breaks should be taken often, especially after a success.

If the student is experiencing difficulty, or overwhelming confusion and disorientation, a break from the activity is a must. It is usually a sure indication that an environmental, physical or emotional distraction is present, or that an earlier confusion or disorientation was overlooked. Be sure to find out which, and remedy the cause before continuing.

Techniques that can also facilitate this process are:

1. The helper does the exercises and clay representations along with the student.
2. The student instructs or tests the helper in the materials just covered.
3. The helper takes turns with the student making up example sentences and usage examples.

The materials you will need are:

- 2 pounds of Plastelina clay per person
- Examples of upper- and lowercase alphabets (enlarge the examples on pages 222 and 223 as a model)
- Dictionary
- Grammar book
- Primers, readers, workbooks, magazines and other reading materials
- Paper

- Pencil
- Tools for cutting and shaping the clay
- Cleanup materials: paper towels or baby wipes

The End of the "Alphabet Song"

After Orientation Counseling (or Alignment), Symbol Mastery is used to master the alphabet and punctuation.

We use a basic form of Symbol Mastery for letters and symbols. The process is simple; we just want the person to master the symbols so they no longer trigger disorientations. We have him create each symbol in modeling clay, identify it and learn its use. For the alphabet, we have him create each letter. We start with the uppercase letters, working from *A* to *Z*.

Alphabet Mastery Procedure

1. Familiarize the person with clay. Shaping. Cutting. Rolling.
2. At any sign of disorientation, always stop, and politely say: "Check your orientation," "Get your dot/dots," or "Feel your imaginary hands." Then resume.
3. Have the person make the uppercase alphabet letters *A* to *Z* in forward order. Letters should be at least two inches high. Written examples

of the letters should be nearby for visual reference (see illustration).

4. Ask the person "Whose alphabet is this?" Repeat the question conversationally until the person says, "It's mine." Then ask the person, "Why?" or "How come?" until the person says, "Because I made it" or "Because I created it."

5. Have the person check to see that all the letters are correctly positioned and sequenced, and similar in size. If any errors are found, have the person compare with the examples and correct them.

   Note: When doing Symbol Mastery, never:
   - criticize the person's artistic ability
   - point out specific mistakes (Have the person check orientation/alignment, then compare his or her clay alphabet with the printed example.)

6. Ask the person, "Are you happy with your alphabet?" If not, ask what could be better, and have him correct it until he is happy with it.

7. Ask the person how many letters are in the alphabet. If he isn't sure, have him count them (slowly). Repeat this activity until the person is absolutely certain there are 26.

8. Have the person slowly and deliberately touch and say the name of each letter in forward order.

9. Have the person touch and say the name of each letter in backward order, starting from Z.

10. Note any errors, hesitations and confusions.

11. When two letters cause confusion or get mixed up, ask the person:

    A. "Tell me something similar about these two letters."

    B. "Tell me something different about these two letters."

    Alternate asking questions A and B until there are no more answers.

    For sequential errors or omissions, ask (with person looking at the letter):

    - A. "What letter comes before ___?"
    - B. "What letter comes after ___?"

12. Have the person touch and say the letters forward and backward. Repeat until it becomes easy.

13. Have the person say the alphabet forward, looking at the letters as needed.

14. Call out a letter of the alphabet, and have the person touch and say what letter comes before and after that letter. Do this until the person can easily and quickly find any letter in the alphabet.

15. Have the person say the alphabet backward, taking as many "peeks" as needed to get through it. Again, look for letters that cause problems, repeated looks and repeated confusions. Check for orientation,

A B C D E F G H I
J K L M N O P Q R
S T U V W X Y Z

Here are the upper- and lowercase letters used for Alphabet Mastery at the Davis Dyslexia Correction Center. They were specially designed for modeling in clay. Enlarge these pages by about 150 percent on a photocopier, then cut each copy into three strips. Tape them together to make long strips that look like these:

A B C D E F G H I J K L M N O P Q R S T U V W X Y Z

zyxwvvutsrqponmlkjihgfedcba

zyxwvuts
rqponmlkji
hgfedcba

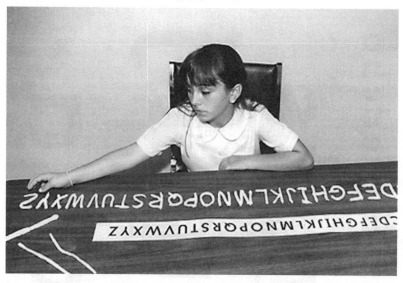

Touch and say the letters in both directions.

and apply step 11 to these letters as needed. Do this until the person can say the whole alphabet backward at least once without looking.

16. If any signs of struggling or frustration appear, *back off* from this task. Take a short break. Then check orientation and go back to the step just preceding the one where trouble occurred. Repeat that step to a new success.

17. Continue to practice the alphabet backward and forward until the person knows it and can easily and comfortably recite it in both directions. Praise lavishly when this is accomplished. Always take a good break after this accomplishment.

18. Have the person make the alphabet in lowercase script backward, *z* through *a*, in reverse order (but not with reversed letters). Use the examples at the beginning of this chapter.

19. As above, monitor for problem letters, check orientation as needed, and have the person check for accuracy.

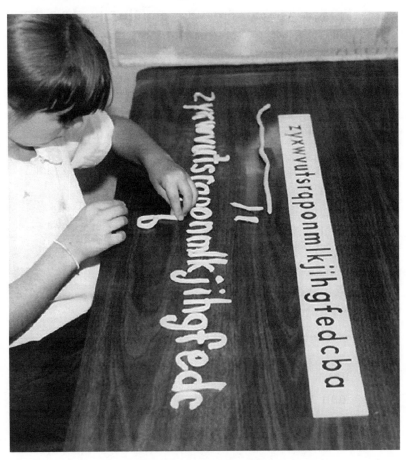

Lowercase letters are made in reverse order.

20. Have the person touch and say the letters in backward order, *z* through *a*.

21. Now have the person recite the alphabet forward. Watch for any signs of the "Alphabet Song," and slow the person down to say each letter separately and distinctly.

22. Randomly selecting any letter, ask the person what letter comes before and after it. Have the person peek, as needed, until he can comfortably tell you what letters come before and after every letter of the alphabet at random without looking.

Additional Exercises That Could Be Done Here or Later

- Finding capital letters in the environment and naming them
- Finding letter sections in the dictionary
- Identifying letters in books
- Finding letter sections in file cabinets, phone books, encyclopedias, etc.
- Noticing different print styles and typefaces
- Writing the letters

The work with the alphabet is complete when the person can recite the alphabet forward and backward with equal ease and speed, and can tell what letters come before and after every letter in the alphabet. At this point, he knows the alphabet well enough not to be dependent on the "Alphabet Song." There is no longer any need to sing it mentally, so the habit will disappear.

Next, we have the person go through the punctuation symbols. At first, it is more important for the dyslexic to know what to *do* when the marks are seen when reading aloud than to know how they are used in writing. This can be covered later.

Punctuation Marks Mastery

1. Go over the definition of "punctuation" from a simple dictionary.
2. Have the person make the period with clay.
3. Have the person write or copy the name of the mark on a small piece of paper (about 4 x 4 inches) and place the clay mark on the piece of paper in proper spatial relation to what they have written. This can become a creative game. Here are a few examples:

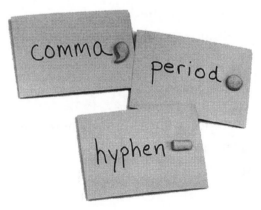

4. Point out the mark in various texts such as a primer, magazine, sign, etc. Also point out how the shape differs depending upon print style or typeface.

5. Have the student find the mark in various texts.

6. Referring to a grammar book or dictionary definition, go over the common usage of each mark. Emphasize what the person should *do* when he sees the mark while reading aloud. Stop for periods, pause for commas, lilt the voice for question marks, etc.

7. Have the student give verbal or written examples of how each punctuation mark is used.

8. Be sure the person knows how to pronounce the name of each mark.

9. Repeat steps 2 to 8 with the:

> Question mark
> Exclamation mark
> Comma
> Apostrophe
> Dash
> Hyphen
> Quotation marks: double and single
> Parentheses
> Brackets

Ellipsis
Asterisk
Colon
Semicolon
Virgule or Slash

Because words are symbols that represent both sound and meaning, it is important that the person also be coached through all the speech sounds. This doesn't require a speech therapist, only the pronunciation key from any dictionary and a good coach.

If numbers are triggers for a person, the same basic process is done with numbers. All of these basic symbols and steps should completed before the Trigger Word list is started.

Additional Symbol Mastery Exercises

Pronunciation Mastery

1. Using a pronunciation key in a dictionary, demonstrate and practice how each of the letters is pronounced and made by the mouth, lips and tongue.
2. Clarify each of the various symbols (diacritical marks) used in the pronunciation key, one at a time, using many examples.

3. Be sure to clarify the *schwa* sound and symbol.
4. Clarify what syllables are, then practice finding them and counting them in some different words.
5. Clarify the use of accents and the accent symbols.
6. Find a word in a dictionary that the person has no idea how to pronounce. Have the person figure out how to pronounce it using the pronunciation key—one syllable at a time, accenting correctly.

Print Styles and Typefaces

1. Using various texts, or ideally a book of printer's typefaces, point out some differences between the letters and numbers of varying typefaces.
2. Have the person find and point out some differences.
3. Have the person note the differences between the following:
   - lowercase *a, g, q, t* and *y* from one print style and another
   - uppercase *I* and lower case *l*
   - letters with and without serifs
4. Be alert for disorientations, and always have the person correct them.
5. If needed, have the person make different types of letters in clay, and note similarities and differences.

6. Good examples and sources of differing print styles are computer fonts, phone book Yellow Pages, cartoon lettering, and newspaper and magazine advertisements.

Other Symbols

Math, scientific, measurement, musical and other symbols that trigger disorientations can be addressed, clarified and mastered in the same manner as above.

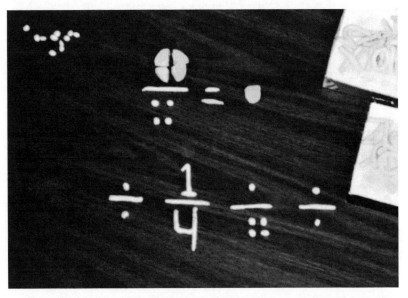

An example of how Symbol Mastery is used to represent the math concept of the fraction ¼.

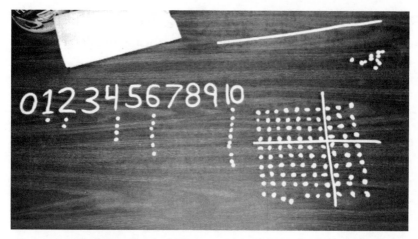

An example of how Symbol Mastery is used to show the meaning of the numerals 1, 2, 4, 6 and 10, and the concept of 7 x 4 = 28.

First-Grade Stuff

Dan, who came for Orientation Counseling between his freshman and sophomore years in high school, had an attitude typical of many dyslexic teenagers. He projected an air of exaggerated self-confidence and made the most of his natural ability to talk a blue streak. He could have become a great salesman even if he had never done anything about his learning disability.

His initial Orientation Counseling session went well, and it was easy for him to maintain his orientation.

When we asked him to construct a clay alphabet, he had the same reaction as so many adults and teenagers: "This is first-grade stuff!" He grumbled, but he went through the basic Symbol Mastery exercises and learned the alphabet backward and forward.

The first word from the trigger word list he chose to master was *the*. To show the definition, he made a ball of clay and a model of a person pointing at it. Suddenly his face flushed, and his eyes began to tear up. He slammed his fist down on the table and said, "Damn! Why didn't they teach me this in first grade? It's so simple!"

"I guess they just didn't know how" was the best answer I could come up with.

CHAPTER 34

Three Steps to Easier Reading

Dyslexic Perception and Certainty

Because dyslexics' attention and awareness are widely spread out around the environment, they will naturally *look* at a word the same way they look at a tree in the park. They will see the entire tree at once. They don't first see the leaves on the left side, then the branches, then the trunk, then the branches and leaves on the right side. They just see the whole tree.

When dyslexics learn to read while looking at entire words, they will always be guessing at what each word is, based on its overall appearance. Guessing will prevent the feeling of certainty they need to gain confidence in their reading ability.

These simple exercises were developed to enable nonreaders to learn the most basic skills needed for comfortable reading, and to help dyslexics learn to read with ease and comprehension.

234

These reading exercises should be used only after the person has completed both Alphabet Mastery and Punctuation Marks Mastery as described in chapter 33.

Begin using these exercises when the person starts to do Symbol Mastery on the Trigger Word list (see chapter 35). It helps to vary the schedule and switch tasks occasionally. This prevents boredom.

1. Spell-Reading

The purposes of Spell-Reading are as follows:

1. To train the person in left to right eye movement in reading
2. To enable the person to recognize letter groups as words

A Spell-Reading session should be limited to a maximum of ten minutes, with breaks of the same length between sessions.

At this point, the person's understanding of what he reads is of no concern. Your goal is only to get the person to recognize the letters in a word and then to repeat the word after you. This is not a phonics or a phonetic process, it is simply letter and word recognition. If the person has had previous instruction in sounding out words and attempts to do this, simply say, "You don't need to sound out the word. Only say the name of the letters one at a time. All we want is for you to name

235

the alphabet letters in the order they're written. Then you say the word after I say it."

The Procedure

Spell-Reading trains the person's brain and eyes to scan from left to right while reading. Just as a computer must receive data in a proper sequence, the brain of the dyslexic needs the data in the order it was meant to be read. The proper sequence for reading in most languages is from left to right. Of course, this procedure also can be adapted for learning to scan the lines of a second language that is arranged from right to left, or from top to bottom.

Dyslexics commonly have two reading habits that limit their ability:

1. Trying to go too fast
2. "Working too hard" by concentrating heavily on the reading material

These can be eliminated by Spell-Reading.

Before starting each session, tell the person, "I want you to go slow and easy. Being sure of what you're reading is more important than going fast. Going slow and easy will make this easy for you."

Also, you want the person to maintain orientation while Spell-Reading. Whenever a person makes an error or shows signs of concentration, have him check orientation. Just say, "Check your point" or "Get your hands."

Adults vs. Children

With a child, use a primer or first-grade reader for the process. Doing Spell-Reading with an adult works the same, but you'll need reading material that won't seem demeaning to the person. Use a simple text like this book or a newspaper. Even though this may be more difficult at first, there will be a bigger boost in self-esteem once the challenge is overcome.

Getting Started

Be sure the environment is comfortable and adequately lit for the person.

How the words are presented can vary, depending on the person's skill level. Most people can scan from one word to the next on a printed page. Others may be overwhelmed by the number of words they see at once. In this case, use a piece of paper to cover everything below the line the person is reading. Then use a second piece of paper to cover the right section of the line you are working on, so each word (or letter) can be revealed one at a time by sliding the paper from left to right.

Sit across from the person with the reading material on the table between you. At the beginning of the session, tell the person: "You spell the word letter by letter. Then I will say the word. Then you say the word. If you suddenly know what the word is while you are spelling it, finish spelling it, then go ahead and say it without waiting for me."

Present the words, letter by letter, by pointing them out with your finger or a pencil, or revealing the words, letter by letter, with sheets of paper as described above.

Insist that the person go slow and easy.

It is your responsibility to catch the person's disorientations. Watch out for:

- Substitution, omission or alteration of a letter
- Moving the head closer to the page
- Speech changes, such as hesitation, speeding up, slowing down or reading in a flat, monotone voice
- Rubbing the neck, fidgeting or wrinkling the eyebrows

At the first sign of any disorientation, cover the material with your hand and ask the person to check orientation or alignment. If need be, take a short break.

Praise any and all improvement. Your praise is the person's reward. It will lift the person's self-esteem.

During this exercise, a point will be reached when the person recognizes many words while spelling them, or even before beginning to spell them. At this point, advance to the Sweep-Sweep-Spell Exercise.

2. Sweep-Sweep-Spell

The purpose of Sweep-Sweep-Spell is to continue training in left-right eye movement and word recognition. Understanding what is read is *not* the goal yet. If you have been revealing the words rather than pointing them out, have the person slide the pieces of paper to reveal individual words and lines of text. As the person improves in the skills of word recognition and eye movement, get rid of the piece of paper that is slid left to right, and slide only one piece of paper down the page to reveal an entire line at a time.

The new instruction is: "Let your eyes sweep through (or over) the word. If the word doesn't just come out of your mouth, sweep it again. If it doesn't come out of your mouth the second time, spell it. Then I'll tell you what it is, and you repeat it."

At the first sign of any disorientation, cover the material with your hand and ask the person to check orientation or alignment.

Sincerely praise each sign of improvement.

If you are working with a child using a primer or first-grade reader, use this step until most of the words are recognized while sweeping them. Then say, "This book is too easy. We need to use something harder." Increase the difficulty of the material one grade level at a time. At first, the person may have some doubt or reservation about reading something harder. Say, "If it's too hard, we can always come back."

When the person can recognize almost every word at the person's appropriate grade level, switch to the next reading exercise: Picture-at-Punctuation.

3. Picture-at-Punctuation

The only purpose of reading is understanding what is read. Reading without full and complete comprehension of what is read is the source of most misunderstanding in any subject at any level.

The goal of Picture-at-Punctuation is full and complete comprehension of what is read.

In Western written languages, each complete thought is either followed by or surrounded (bracketed) by punctuation marks. Each complete thought can be either pictured or felt.

Tell the person, "We are now going to add meaning to what you're reading. To us, punctuation means 'picture.' When you see a punctuation mark, make a picture in your mind of what you just read."

Picture-at-Punctuation is an added step to Sweep-Sweep-Spell.

Point out the punctuation marks where the person should stop and form a mental picture:

- Periods
- Exclamation marks
- Question marks

- Commas
- Quotation marks
- Semicolons
- Dashes
- Parentheses or brackets
- Colons

Have the person read a short sentence or part of a sentence (only the words leading up to the first punctuation mark). Stop the person from looking at the words just read. Cover the words with your hand if you need to.

Ask the person, "What do you see?"

If the part of a sentence is something that cannot be pictured, like "long ago," or "once upon a time," ask, "What do you feel?" or "What does that mean to you?"

Sometimes you will encounter non-trigger words or unknown words for which the person simply has no meaning. When this happens, you can explain the meaning of the word or look it up in a simple dictionary.

Some trigger words will cause disorientations. Point out that the word is a Trigger Word. Say "check your point" or "get your hands" and, once done, pick up where the disorientation occurred. If they have already done Symbol Mastery on that word, you have hit a particular definition of the word that will also need to be mastered.

At some point, the person will start reading voluntarily for pleasure. Once you notice that someone is reading articles simply because they're interesting, your job is done. Do more coaching only if it is requested, and encourage the person to use Symbol Mastery for any words or expressions that cause confusion.

CHAPTER 35

Symbol Mastery for Words

Most people, including those without dyslexia, don't know the definitions of the common trigger words, even though they happen to be the most frequently used words in the English language. I have met English teachers who couldn't define *a* or *the* as other than "articles." Anyone's reading skill and comprehension will be vastly improved by mastering the definitions of these words.

No Concentration Allowed

Symbol Mastery should be a playful, game-like activity. Consider that the words and symbols are little puzzles, with each definition forming a piece of the puzzle. Most dyslexics have had frustrating experiences in school, so many rely on rote memorization to give the appearance of learning something. Building the forms of the letters in clay not only helps break the habit of heavy concentration, but allows the person to do something creative as a learning activity.

Whether you are doing Symbol Mastery by yourself or helping someone else with it, make it a true learning experience. Make it OK to make mistakes and get things wrong sometimes. Finding mistakes is one of the best ways to learn things. Very few people have already studied or know all the definitions of these words.

If the person gets stumped on a particular word or symbol, just mark it for future reference and go on to one that is easy. If the going gets tedious, take a break, do Release and check for orientation.

Following is the Davis Symbol Mastery procedure for words, some hints on getting started and the list of Trigger Words.

Symbol Mastery Procedure

1. Look up the word in a dictionary or glossary.
2. If you don't know how to pronounce it, find out.
3. Read the first definition and example sentences aloud.
4. Establish a clear understanding of the definition. Discuss it. Make up sentences or phrases using the word with that definition. Do this until you have a clear picture of this definition in your mind.

5. Make a clay model of the concept described by the definition. How to make a clay model is described in the hints below.

6. Make the symbol or the letters of the word out of clay. Make sure the word is spelled correctly. Use lowercase letters unless the word is a proper noun that is normally capitalized.

7. Make a mental picture of what has been created.

8. Say aloud to the model: "You are (word), meaning (definition)."

   (Example: "You are *tall*, meaning *of more than normal height*.")

9. Say aloud to the word or symbol: "You say (word)."

   (Example: "You say *tall*.")

Make up more sentences and phrases until you can do so easily. Be sure the usage of the word matches the definition you just made.

These additional exercises are optional:

- Touch and say the letters of the word
- Write the word

Before diving into the Trigger Words, practice the steps of Symbol Mastery on some common word such as *lamb*, *apple* or *cat*. Nouns tend to be easy to picture and make in clay. After that, try a verb or adjective such as *jump* or *tall*. This will get the person used to doing each of the steps.

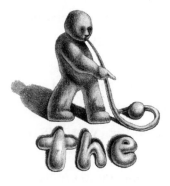

the

1. that which is here or which has been mentioned *[Give me the ball. Open the book.]*

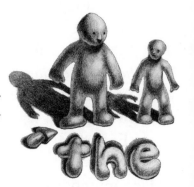

2. that one of a number or group *[The man on the left is taller. Take the one on top.]*

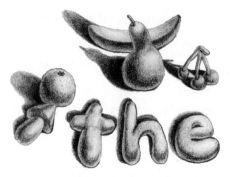

3. any one of a certain kind *[The orange is a fruit. The elephant is a mammal.]*

*Examples of how three definitions of the word "the"
can be represented with Symbol Mastery.*

Depending on the individual, there may be additional Trigger Words besides those listed below that need to be mastered. These could be key words in a difficult subject, words that are consistently misspelled, homonyms, new vocabulary or words that are repeatedly misread. Just note them as they are encountered and add them to the list of words that need to be mastered.

Symbol Mastery Hints for Trigger Words

The trigger words listed below are those that most often cause confusion and disorientation when reading, writing or communicating. They are confusing because:

a. The person does not have a mental image of what the word means or represents.

b. Many of these words have multiple meanings.

Here are ways to make mastering them easier:

1. Use a dictionary that gives example sentences or phrases along with each definition.

2. Make up example sentences and phrases with a particular definition until you are sure you know it, are comfortable using the word with that definition and can easily imagine a clay model that would fully show the definition in your mind.

3. Start with words that have only a few definitions, such as the articles *a, an* and *the*, and the pronouns *I, you, me, we, him, her, this* and *that.*

4. Substitute the definition for the word itself in a phrase or sentence. This helps clarify the meaning so you'll know if you are using the word correctly.

Example

The word *a* can mean "one" or "for each." If you are doing the first definition, where it means "one," and your sentence is "Eggs are $1.00 *a* dozen," you can substitute the definition "one" for the word *a* in your sentence. "Eggs are $1.00 *one* dozen" doesn't sound right or make sense. Using the other definition "for each," the substitution would be "Eggs are $1.00 *for each* dozen," which is correct.

---

5. Master the first or major definition of each word on the list first, and create only two to four definitions per session. Doing too many definitions at once will cause confusion. Once you have completed the first or major definition of all the words, go through the list again and complete the rest of the definitions for each word.

6. If you hit a definition you can't make sense of, there is probably a word *within the definition itself* that is another Trigger Word. You can look up these words and master them, or look in another dictionary to see if it explains that particular definition more clearly.

7. The word *be* and its other forms, such as *is*, *was* and *are*, are the most difficult words on the list to master. Save them for last, and have a grammar book handy.

8. Make sure the clay figures and models you make are "realistic." This does not mean they have to be extremely artistic or exactly lifelike. It means they should be three-dimensional and should represent physical reality in a recognizable way. They should not be overly abstract or symbolic. A blob of clay cannot be representative of a car; the blob must at least have four wheels!

9. A clay model of a person can be made to look like a stick figure, but it should be large enough and sturdy enough to stand on its own. When you need to show action or emotion, it needs arms and legs that can be positioned and a head that can have facial expressions carved into it.

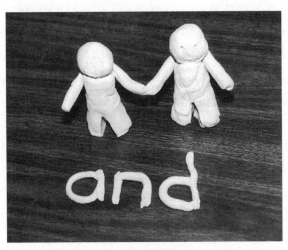

A child's model of the definition of "and."

10. Use clay arrows to show directions or sequence.

11. Make a clay rope into a "cartoon bubble" that is attached to a person's head to show that something is an idea or is happening in the mind. Show what is going on in the mind within the borders of the bubble. Speech can be shown the same way.

12. Make the clay letters of the words in lowercase "printed" form, the way they most often appear in books. Only *I* and other proper names are always capitalized. Check to see that you have spelled the word correctly after you have made it out of clay.

13. Some words are grouped with their different tenses and forms. You should use a grammar book to fully understand them. This is an opportunity to learn and master what happens to a word when you add different endings to it such as *-ed*, *-s* and *-ing*, and also how words can change depending on whether you are talking about the present, the past or the future.

14. As you progress through the words, you may notice that the definitions of each word are grouped according to what kind of word they are (parts of speech: noun, adjective, adverb, verb, pronoun, conjunction, preposition or interjection). Looking in a grammar book and learning what these are can help make the differences between the definitions clearer.

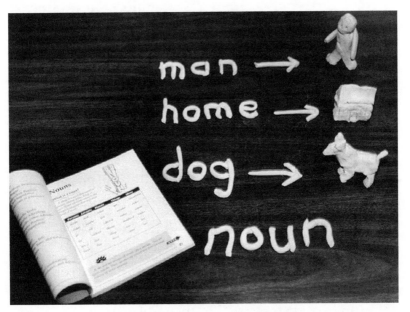

A clay model of the word "noun."

15. If a definition seems hard or confusing, take a brief break. Look out a window, stand up for a minute or just stretch your arms, and be sure to check orientation before continuing.

The Trigger Words

The Key Triggers for Disorientation

NOTE: *Words with more than one form are in* **boldface** *type,*
followed by their other forms.

a	*was*	**do**	*got*
about	*were*	*did*	**go**
again	*being*	*does*	*goes*
ago	*been*	*doing*	*going*
all	*because*	*done*	*gone*
almost	**become**	*don't*	**have**
also	*became*	*doesn't*	*had*
always	*becoming*	*down*	*has*
an	*becomes*	*each*	*having*
and	*before*	*either*	*he*
another	*between*	*else*	*he's*
any	*but*	*even*	*her*
anyhow	*by*	*ever*	*hers*
anyway	**can**	*every*	*here*
as	*could*	*everything*	*him*
at	*can't*	*for*	*his*
away	*cannot*	*from*	*how*
back	**come**	*front*	*I*
be	*came*	*full*	*if*
am	*comes*	**get**	*in*
are	*coming*	*gets*	*into*
is	*could*	*getting*	*isn't*

it	*more*	*ran*	*the*
its	*most*	*running*	*their*
it's	*much*	*runs*	*theirs*
just	*my*	*same*	*them*
last	*neither*	**see**	*then*
leave	*never*	*saw*	*there*
leaves	*no*	*seen*	*there's*
leaving	*none*	*sees*	*these*
least	*nor*	*she*	*they*
left	*not*	*she's*	*they're*
less	*now*	*shall*	*this*
let	*of*	*should*	*those*
lets	*off*	*so*	*through*
let's	*on*	*some*	*to*
letting	*one*	*soon*	*too*
like	*onto*	**stand**	*unless*
liked	*or*	*standing*	*until*
likes	*other*	*stands*	*up*
liking	*others*	*stood*	*upon*
make	*otherwise*	*such*	*us*
made	*our*	*sure*	*very*
makes	*ours*	**take**	*we*
making	*out*	*takes*	*we're*
many	*over*	*taking*	*what*
may	**put**	*took*	*when*
maybe	*puts*	*than*	*where*
me	*putting*	*that*	*where's*
mine	**run**	*that's*	*whether*

which	why	won't	you're
while	will	would	yours
who	with	yet	
who's	within	you	
whose	without	your	

CHAPTER 36

Continuing the Process

The purpose of taking someone through the procedures described in the previous chapters is to correct the learning disability aspect of dyslexia.

The Davis Dyslexia Correction Program offered by Davis Facilitators takes an average of 30 hours. Most of that time is devoted to Symbol Mastery of the person's own unique triggering symbols. Our job is to train people in the skills for controlling their orientation and help them to master the Symbol Mastery technique. Fully mastering the words on the Trigger Words List is their assignment after completing our program. Training for a parent, spouse or other family member is included in the program so that support can continue at home. People who go through a professional program can also come back for one or more short "tune-up" sessions.

The task of correction isn't really complete until the

person's compulsive solutions no longer operate. As long as the person continues to use the old solutions, he might as well keep the old problem, because nothing will permanently change. So in order for dyslexia to be corrected, the old, compulsive solutions simply have to go.

The entire sequence of events that resulted in the person acquiring an old solution in the first place began because the person couldn't think with a written symbol or trigger word. Mastering just the first or primary definition of a trigger word will allow the person to begin to think with that word nonverbally. That word will cease to cause an old solution to occur. As each word is mastered—even partially—the old solutions will fade away on their own.

The old solutions are no longer stimulated, so they don't automatically happen. As the person experiences life, he or she will discover things that work better than the old solutions did. As soon as the person experiences a better way of doing things, the old solutions are replaced.

The idea that deeply embedded compulsive behaviors could simply fall away on their own may sound incredible, but they do, especially in a patient, supportive environment. After a few months, most of them should disappear.

Experiencing the loss of an old solution is all the proof a person needs in order to know with certainty that his dyslexia is being corrected, and that the change is permanent.

This isn't to say dyslexics should master only the first or primary definitions of trigger words. That is when the old solutions begin to disappear, but a word isn't truly mastered until all of its definitions are mastered. Dyslexics should exercise their *gift of mastery* and really get the job done thoroughly.

The person should also remember to check orientation whenever disorientation occurs for any reason. There will be things other than words in the person's life or environment that stimulate disorientation. These spontaneous disorientations aren't dyslexia, but they do share the same characteristics. They can often cause phobias. Orientation turns them *off*. However, fully dealing with phobias is not the subject of this book.

The person should also continue to master confusing words as they are encountered, using the Symbol Mastery Procedure. It's a great way to study new subjects. In fact, for many corrected dyslexics attending colleges and universities, simply mastering the words in the glossaries of textbooks with this process has enabled them to achieve a 3.0 or better grade point average.

The final thought I want to leave you with is something I said at the end of chapter 21.

*W*hen someone
masters something,
it becomes a part
of that person.
It becomes part of
the individual's thought
and creative process.
It adds the quality of
its essence to all
subsequent thought
and creativity of
the individual.

Ronald D. Davis
The Gift of Dyslexia

*Note: This page is exempt from copyright.
Feel free to enlarge it on your copier.*

258

Recommended References

Dictionaries

Webster's New World Children's Dictionary
Macmillan
Clearly written, well formatted and nicely illustrated, this dictionary is excellent for doing Symbol Mastery with all age groups. Included with the Davis Symbol Mastery kit (see order form).

The Concise Oxford Dictionary of Current English
Oxford University Press
Although you might need a magnifying glass, when it comes to the Queen's English, there is no better reference. This is where you will find literary or obscure definitions for a word.

The World Book Dictionary
World Book–Childcraft International
For the person who gets addicted to Symbol Mastery or learns to love words, this two-volume dictionary is one of the best.

Grammar and Writing Improvement

Terban, Marvin
Checking Your Grammar
Scholastic Inc.
A simple, concise presentation of all the basic elements of grammar, with lots of examples. Indexed. Included with the Davis Symbol Mastery Kit (see order form).

Recommended Reading

Armstrong, Thomas, PhD
The Myth of the ADD Child
Dutton
Dr. Armstrong presents 50 strategies parents can use to improve children's behavior and attention span without drugs, labels or coercion.

Davis, Ronald D.
The Gift of Learning: Proven New Methods for Correcting ADD, Math and Handwriting Problems
Perigee
Provides innovative theory and detailed instructions for the Davis approach to resolving attention focus, math and handwriting difficulties.

Freed, Jeffrey, and Laurie Parsons
Right-Brained Children in a Left-Brained World: Unlocking the Potential of Your ADD Child

Fireside
This book offers a step-by-step program that shows parents how to work with, rather than against, the special abilities of the ADD child.

Hartmann, Thom
Attention Deficit Disorder: A Different Perception
Underwood Books
Explores the benefits of the ADD mind, and provides good reasons for "distractible" people to celebrate their creative thinking style.

Marshall, Abigail
The Everything Parents Guide to Children with Dyslexia
Adams Media
This book provides practical advice to parents, an overview of different teaching methods and treatment programs for dyslexia, and helpful tips and suggestions for helping children with schoolwork.

Smith, Joan
You Don't Have to Be Dyslexic
Learning Time Products
Dr. Smith describes assessment and treatment procedures that have proven success helping dyslexic children and adults. Clearly written and narrated with numerous case histories.

West, Thomas G.
In the Mind's Eye
Prometheus Books
An in-depth look at the connections between creative ability, visual thinking, academic learning difficulties and the remarkable people who share these traits.

Recorded Books

Recording for the Blind and Dyslexic
20 Roszel Road
Princeton, NJ 08540
(609) 452-0606
www.rfbd.org
This organization recently changed its name to incorporate people with "word blindness" (an earlier term for dyslexia). Their extended-play tapes require a special player. More than 75,000 educational and professional books are available, including school textbooks and *The Gift of Dyslexia.*

Davis Resource Sites

www.dyslexia.com
Information about Davis workshops, public lectures, recommended books and materials, and qualified Davis Facilitators in over 40 nations, providing Davis Programs in over 30 languages.

www.dyslexiatalk.com
Online support forum for parents, teachers and dyslexic adults.

www.davisautism.com
Information about the Davis Autism Approach Program for enabling individuals with autism, PDD and Asperger syndrome to fully participate in life.

www.davislearn.com
Information for teachers and school administrators about the Davis Learning and Strategies program for enhancing the learning skills of all children in primary level classrooms.

www.thedyslexicreader.org
Archived copies of *The Dyslexic Reader* newsletter.

Dyslexia support organisations in the UK

The British Dyslexia Association (BDA)
A national charity whose vision is a dyslexia friendly society enabling all dyslexic people to reach their potential. BDA works with parents, teachers and health care professionals.

The British Dyslexia Association
Unit 8 Bracknell Beeches
Old Bracknell Lane
Bracknell RG12 7BW

National helpline: 0845 251 9002

http://www.bdadyslexia.org.uk

Dyslexia Action
A national educational charity who provide help and support for people with dyslexia and literacy difficulties. Dyslexia Action offer a wide range of teaching resources and support across the UK.

Dyslexia Action
Park House
Wick Road
Egham TW20 0HH

Telephone: 01784 222 300

http://www.dyslexiaaction.org.uk

Glossary

Acalculia: an inability to develop mathematical skills. *A person with acalculia cannot do arithmetic.*

ADD: acronym and abbreviation for attention deficit disorder. *ADD is described in* The Merck Manual of Diagnosis and Therapy.

Agraphia: an inability to manipulate a writing instrument or express thoughts in writing. *A person with agraphia may speak well but cannot write.*

Alignment: a Davis Orientation Counseling procedure that resolves disorientation and ensures accurate perception for individuals who are primarily kinesthetic or tactile learners. *We check Alignment with our balance.*

Alphabet: the letters of a language in their customary order. *The English alphabet has 26 letters.*

Attention: awareness of the environment. *Attention is what is used when enjoying a beautiful sunset.*

Attention Deficit Disorder: *see ADD.*

Balance: ability to stand on one foot without wobbling; a perception that can be used to check orientation. *By checking our balance we can tell if we are oriented.*

Concentration: limiting one's awareness to only one thing. *Heavy concentration produces a hypnotic state.*

Concept: an idea or thought; a mental picture; an idea of what something is, or what a group of things are. *Words are used to communicate a concept.*

Conceptualization: an image, idea, thought or concept that is created in the mind; the act of mentally creating something. *Conceptualization occurs in the mind.*

Confusion: an overwhelming feeling of blankness. *Confusion causes disorientation in dyslexics.*

Counseling: helping people improve their abilities or get rid of their disabilities. *We get counseling when we need help with a problem.*

Davis Dyslexia Correction Program: an individualized counseling program where a person learns how to correct disorientations, maintain orientation and improve reading, writing, math or attention focus skills. *The Davis Dyslexia Correction Program takes about 30 hours to complete.*

Davis Orientation Counseling: procedures that help a person create, find and use a stable location for the mind's eye; methods for controlling, monitoring and turning off disorientations. *Davis Orientation Counseling shows a person how to self-correct disorientations.*

Davis Symbol Mastery: a procedure for learning what a symbol means, what it looks like and what it sounds like. *We create concepts with clay when we do Davis Symbol Mastery.*

Definition: a statement that tells the meaning of a word. *Tell me the definition of that word.*

Disorient: to lose one's position or direction in relation to the true facts and conditions in the environment; to lose touch with reality to some degree. *People who disorient easily sometimes feel dizzy.*

Disorientation: the loss of one's position or direction in relation to other things; a state of mind in which mental perceptions do not agree with the true facts and conditions in the environment; in some people, this is an automatic response to confusion. *During a disorientation the perceptions are altered.*

Dyscalculia: a form of dyslexia where the difficulty is primarily with math and numbers. A common symptom of dyscalculia is difficulty learning phone numbers.

Dysgraphia: a form of dyslexia where the difficulty is primarily with handwriting. *People with dysgraphia have problems with penmanship.*

Dyslexia: a type of disorientation caused by a natural cognitive ability that can replace normal sensory perceptions with conceptualizations; reading, writing, speaking or directional difficulties that stem from disorientations triggered by confusions regarding symbols. *Dyslexia stems from a perceptual talent.*

Dyspraxia: motor difficulties that can affect body motions. *Dyspraxia can manifest as clumsiness, handwriting problems or speech difficulties.*

Fine Tuning: the Davis procedure for checking and

adjusting orientation using balance. *Fine Tuning improves balance and coordination.*

Holding: the phenomenon of trying to hold the mind's eye in place. *Holding causes headaches.*

Hyperactivity: a condition that can accompany attention deficit disorder where a person appears overly restless, moves about a great deal and can't sit still. *Hyperactivity is the opposite of lethargy.*

Language: speech sounds that have meaning; written symbols that represent speech sounds; the speech and writing of a particular country or group of people. *The only language I know is English.*

Letter: a written symbol that represents a speech sound. *Z is a letter.*

Master: to know with certainty; to practice or do something until it is completely known. *To master something requires practice.*

Mastery: certainty; knowing for sure what something means, looks like or sounds like; knowing how to do something well; knowing without doubt. *His mastery of cooking makes him an excellent chef.*

Meaning: an idea someone has attached to an object or symbol. *All words have a meaning.*

Mind's eye: that which views one's mental images. *The mind's eye is what looks at our imagination.*

Natural orientation: a general location for the mind's eye that naturally occurs with human development. *A* *common natural orientation for a gymnast is several feet straight above the head on midline.*

Nonverbal conceptualization: thinking with mental pictures of concepts or ideas; any form of thinking that does not use words. *Intuition is a form of nonverbal conceptualization.*

"Old solutions": *see Solutions.*

Optimum orientation: placement of the mind's eye that results in all the perceptions being in agreement with each other and accurate; specifically the senses of balance, motion, vision, hearing and time. *Optimum orientation results from Fine Tuning.*

Orient: to put oneself in the proper position and state of mind so one's mental perceptions agree with the true facts and conditions in the environment; to position the mind's eye above and behind the head in a stable location. *When we orient ourselves, we can read better.*

Orientation: putting oneself in the proper position in relation to the true facts and conditions; a state of mind in which mental perceptions agree with the true facts and conditions in the environment. *Orientation makes me feel less confused.*

Orientation point: a stable location above and behind the head (this location varies from person to person). *Put your mind's eye on the orientation point.*

Perception: information that comes to the brain through

the sensory organs and channels. *We determine what is real with our perception.*

Release: a relaxation and stress relief procedure (described in chapter 28). *Do Release when you feel tense.*

Review: a procedure used after Orientation Counseling to check if the orientation point is located in the proper place. *After Fine Tuning, daily Review is unnecessary.*

Solutions (compulsive): behaviors, habits and mental tricks adopted to resolve the mistakes and frustrations caused by disorientation; the components of a learning disability. *Having to sing the "Alphabet Song" is a common solution to not being able to learn the alphabet.*

Stable orientation: a condition in which a person's mind's eye tends to remain in one location most or all of the time. *People who do not experience dyslexic symptoms tend to have a stable orientation.*

Symbol: something that means or represents something else. *The flag is a symbol of our country.*

Threshold for confusion: the point at which the confusion in the environment becomes overwhelming to an individual. *When dyslexics reach their threshold for confusion, they become disoriented.*

Trigger (word): anything that causes disorientation; usually a word or symbol for which a person does not have a complete or accurate concept. *The word "the" is a common trigger word.*

Unstable orientation: a condition in which a person's mind's eye moves about a lot. *People who easily experience motion sickness tend to have an unstable orientation.*

Verbal conceptualization: thinking with the sounds of words. *Hearing your thoughts in words is a form of verbal conceptualization.*

Word: a spoken sound, or letters that represent that sound, which has a meaning or definition in a language. *I learned a new word today.*

Index

Davis Dyslexia Association International

The worldwide organization for Davis training and materials with a searchable database of qualified Davis Facilitators around the world.

1601 Bayshore Highway, Suite 260
Burlingame, CA 94010 USA
Tel: +1 (650) 692-7141 or 1-888-999-3324 (toll-free in USA or Canada)
Fax: +1 (650) 692-7075

International website:
www.dyslexia.com
Professional Training Workshops:
training@dyslexia.com
General inquiries:
ddai@dyslexia.com

United Kingdom

DAVIS DYSLEXIA ASSOCIATION UK
Davis Learning Foundation
47–49 Church Street
Great Malvern
Worcestershire
WR14 2AA

Tel: +44 (0)1684 566300
Email: uk@dyslexia.com
Website: www.davislearningfoundation.org.uk

Australia/New Zealand

DAVIS DYSLEXIA ASSOCIATION PACIFIC
295 Rattray Street
Dunedin
New Zealand 9016

Tel: +64 0274 399 020
Fax: +64 3456 2028
Email: pacific@dyslexia.com
Website: www.davisdyslexia.co.nz

Attention, Readers

The information and methods described in this book are free for all who wish to use them with friends, students and family. However, Davis, Davis Dyslexia Correction, Davis Orientation Counseling, Davis Math Mastery, Davis Attention Mastery, Davis Symbol Mastery, Davis Learning Strategies, Davis Autism Approach, and the DDAI logo are trademarks of Ronald D. Davis and Davis Dyslexia Association International. Use of these marks to represent educational, therapeutic and instructional services or products for sale or commercial purposes is exclusively limited to qualified and licensed professionals who have done extensive training and are required to maintain strict quality standards. When seeking professional help with Davis methods, check with your nearest Davis Dyslexia Association or the website listings at www.dyslexia.com to ensure you are receiving services from a currently certified and licensed Davis Facilitator.